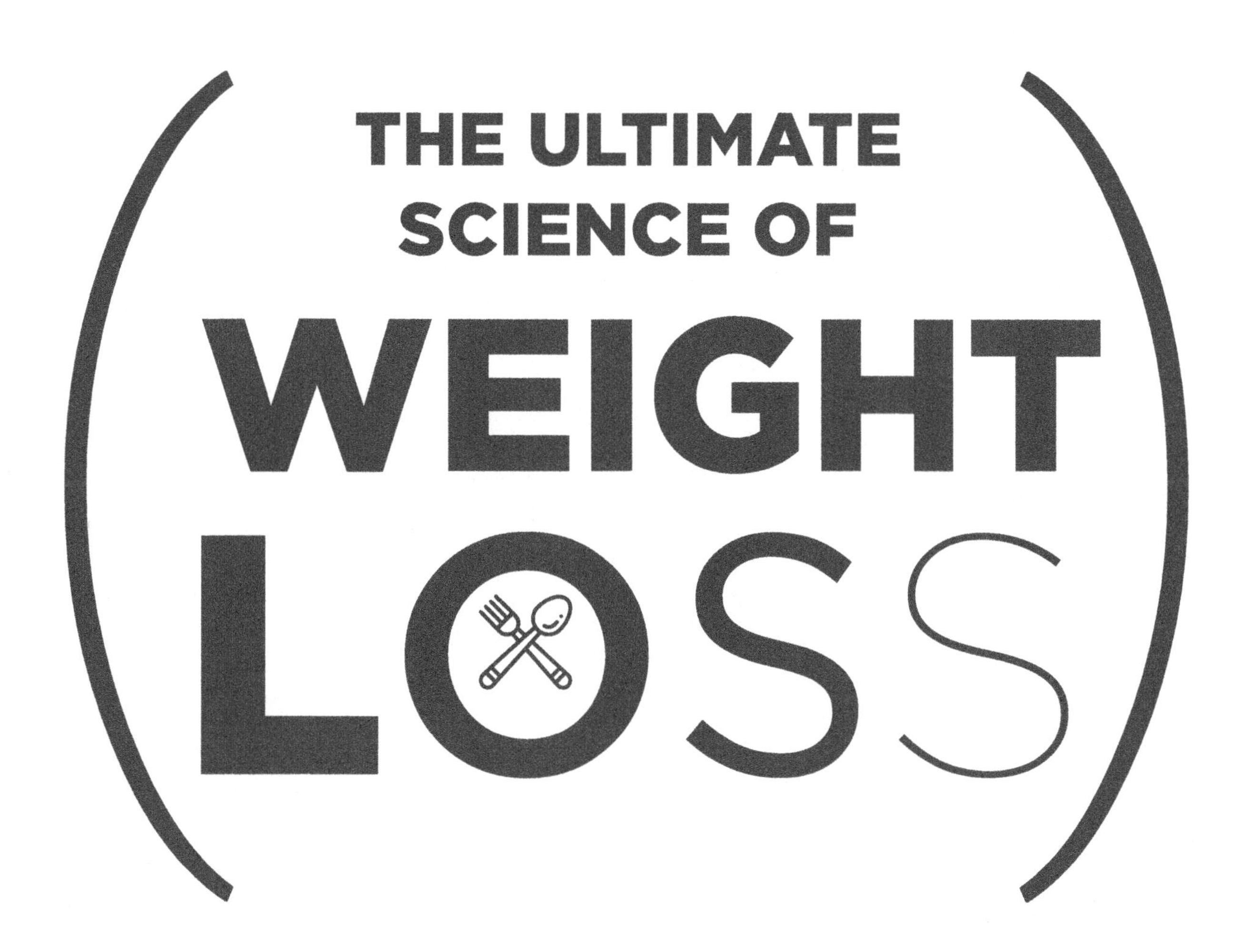

LEARN THE LATEST BREAKTHROUGH DISCOVERIES TO LOSING WEIGHT QUICKLY, EASILY AND PERMANENTLY!

by **Keith Scott-Mumby** MD, MB ChB, HMD, PhD

Published by Mother Whale Inc.
ISBN: 978-0-9913188-8-9

Disclaimer

Managing perfect body weight is not a complicated rocket science. Our body is made up of food which we eat during our day to day life. If we are overweight or obese at the moment then one thing is certain that the food which we eat is unhealthy.

Subodh Gupta

Nothing tastes as good as being thin feels.

Elizabeth Berg

Habit is habit and not to be flung out of the window by any man, but coaxed downstairs a step at a time.

Mark Twain

The groundwork of all happiness is health.

Leigh Hunt

The cardiologist's diet: If it tastes good, spit it out.

Author Unknown

In two decades I've lost a total of 789 pounds. I should be hanging from a charm bracelet.

Erma Bombeck

When we lose twenty pounds... we may be losing the twenty best pounds we have! We may be losing the pounds that contain our genius, our humanity, our love and honesty.

Woody Allen

You have to stay in shape.
My grandmother, she started walking five miles a day when she was 60.
She's 97 today and we don't know where the hell she is.

Ellen Degeneres

CONTENTS

INTRODUCTION

No More Weight Loss Porn!

This is not just another me-too diet book (yawn), but a reasoned and intelligent self-help manual, by a "people's MD", filled with valuable knowledge and helpful TO-DOs. It is actually a lifetime's education in the secrets of up-to-date slimming science; everything you need to know to manage your weight and optimize your health, once and for all.

This is the missing book from the weight loss market. It is packed with information and action strategies for any individual to turn to, for skilled self-management in weight control. This is the final way out of the yo-yo dieting trap.

The shelves at the bookstore are saturated with set diet plans; there are even books on why set diet plans are a bad idea, with titles like *Diets Don't Work* (Bob Schwartz)! We don't need more diet plans. We need public education about overweight and obesity.

Instead of concentrating on suggestions of what to eat and a few recipes for those foods, this milestone book takes the reader beyond, into the realms of revolutionary and recent discoveries in the field of "fat science".

You know the old maxim: give a man a fish and you feed him for a day; but teach a man to fish and you feed him for life. Well, it applies here too. Tell someone what to eat and they lose weight, at least short-term; but teach that person about the role of disturbed bowel flora in causing obesity (could be the number one factor), the influence of fat-bearing genes (there are several), why food allergies and intolerance are major players, the effect of appetite-regulating hormones, ketogenesis, insulin resistance, plus a score of other major discoveries that have a major effect on weight control, and he or she can become truly healthy and remain slim for life.

It's A Game

Slimming, or staying healthy and trim if you are in good shape, is like a game; there are rules. If you don't know these rules, you have little chance of being a winner at the game! Consider this is a book explaining the rules of the game, rather than orchestrated gambits. Learn the rules and you can manage your own success and not rely on others for their understanding or suggestions.

You need to be clear about one thing: very clear. That what you eat is crucial to all aspects of your life and health, not just what you weigh on the bathroom scales. Foods can really hurt you, leading to deteriorating health, feeling weary, organ failure, early death, infertility, impotence, mood swings, unhappiness and a long, long catalogue of similar woes.

Furthermore, the wrong foods that you have been told about over the years are mostly incorrect. The truth is everyone has their own personal "wrong foods" and they are different from person to person.

I have been meaning for some time now to write this book, with an overview of all dieting methods and the science of weight control, as it exists today. It seems to me that I am uniquely suited to do it, since I don't sell or push any particular methods. Plus, I have a far deeper insight into the complex role that allergy foods play in our metabolism than most silly, self-aggrandized "experts", who are just on the make.

The fact that the weight-loss market is a multi-billion dollar market should be an immediate red flag. With that much money on the table (60 billion dollars in 2016 in the USA alone), people are not going to scruple much over what is true or what works, so much as what sells.

This is unfortunate for the would-be dieter. As marketing messages and fashions change, it means ideas come and go that, on the surface, look like something new but in fact are just me-too versions of old and tried ideas. Only the clamor and the claims vary, but that's due to inventiveness and double-talk, not real progress.

There are just a few basic slimming strategies that work; I'll list these in just a moment. The reader will readily see that all successful diets encompass one or more of these simple ideas. It's hard to see how they could be added to. But one must never say "never". One of the most significant revolutions in understanding weight control has come only in recent years and may render all other approaches redundant. I will be giving it considerable emphasis in this book, because I know it's something avoided by most mainstream diet books (bowel flora).

The only thing that doesn't change is that there has to be some change; going on doing the same old thing isn't going to work for you. Mistakes and false foundations lead to blind alleys. Love of burgers or cream buns is great as a food indulgence or a rewarding treat, but will never hack it as a weight loss strategy... not ever!

You have to change.

The Instant NOW Message

One of the vexing trends of modern marketing is to advertise everything as instant. What used to be "90 Days To A Slimmer You" slowly evolved into "How to Lose 30 Pound in 30 Days" to a "7-Day Weight-Loss Diet Meal Plan" to "How To Lose Weight In Less Than 7 Days" to "Instant Weight Loss with The Cabbage Soup Diet" (seriously, I found all these labels offered on the Internet). There is even a "6 day Rapid-Fire Weight Loss Workout", sold on Amazon, presumably just to nudge ahead of the slow crawlers who were taking that extra day!

The trouble is that this craving for instant results, even if it works, ignores the fact that you'll just pile it all back on again, unless you go for a lifelong change of eating habits. You need to learn something, not just hit yourself with avoidance routines.

One of the best diets out there at the time of writing (the Dukan diet) is successful because it isn't a diet; well, at least not *just* a diet. It sensibly includes exercise as part of the program. Movement has to be part of any good health program for one simple reason: we are hard-wired to keep moving.

In Nature, human beings are supposed to be active, nomadic people, wandering through forests and over plains, in search of food and shelter. Constant movement is core to our health and being. Yet we have become so sedentary today that the average person barely walks further than to the bathroom or kitchen; we even have motorized trolleys for riding around in supermarkets!

Being lazy has its attractions (obviously) but it also has inherent dangers. So any suggestion that dieting works without changes in activity levels is just plain nonsense. But you won't see that in most "slimming plans" because to teach exercise is unpopular and the authors don't want the result for you, they want the result for themselves (lots of sales and lots of money). He or she will only sell you what they think you want to hear, instead of what you need to know.

This book is different. You're going to get it between the eyes, whether you are comfortable with the truth or not.

PART 1. THE BASICS

STUFF YOU NEED TO KNOW

PART 1. THE BASICS

SECTION 1. HARD CORE WEIGHT LOSS AND BEYOND

The 4-Phases of Weight Loss

Mireille Guiliano, in her rightly famous book *French Women Don't Get Fat*, suggests a 4-phase view, instead of the craving for instant results. As a lover of French food and drink myself, I think it's worth getting comfortable with her basic plan and not rushing at it.

Phase 1 is educational: spend 3 weeks writing down everything you eat and learn from it. Look for addictions and patterns. What are you actually doing with your diet? What is it that has got you hooked?

Phase 2 is 'recasting': a 3-month stage of being strict and keeping clear of the naughty stuff. Instead, invest the time and effort to learn about food and get some discipline going. It doesn't mean starvation; it does mean intelligence about your eating. This is a good stage in which to learn to cook your own food, if you don't already do so, and get skilled in the kitchen. Gastronomy is a word now associated with good eating but originally meant "the rules of the stomach" (from the Greek).

Three months might seem a long time in contemplation; but as I will be remarking over and over in this book, you only ever have to do it once, if you do it right.

Phase 3 is stabilization: integrating what you have learned into a plan that suits you. By this stage, you should be more than halfway to your target weight and feeling good about your achievements so far. Now you have to re-cast your thoughts to get rid of that "when this is all over" mentality; it's never going to be over. Otherwise you just slob out and get fat again.

However, in phase 3, you will be delighted to learn that you can get away with an occasional teeny indulgence, which is satisfying and enjoyable. Dieting does not have to be misery.

Phase 4 is, quite simply, the rest of your life: You are at or near your target weight, you like your food, you cook in more than you eat out, so you can choose healthy options. By this stage you should have developed healthy habits and if you take care these valuable habits will serve you well. By this stage you will view eating and drinking in a different light; you'll look and feel great; friends will comment and want your advice; you'll be a slimming star!

Moreover, the delight of food should have won you over: delicious, sensuous smells and textures; colors to enhance the taste and lots of freshness and flavor. You won't be eating because you've become addicted to sly ingredients that manufacturers put in their foods (section 2); you'll be eating because it's a real pleasure. You'll enjoy an occasional glass of wine at dinner and even a little chocolate.

There: now did anybody mention sweating and toiling in the gym? Nope!

The Concept Of The Right Diet

So, from the previous section, it is only a small step to introduce my core concept of "the right diet" or "right eating". I cover just about everything about slimming and health here in these pages, so you have got the good and the bad, to help you make wiser choices. But what I most want to get across to you is that *there is a safe, wise and energizing eating pattern that is right for you and you need to find it and adopt it.* It's not the same as other people's best pattern.

Perhaps that idea startles you; you have maybe been indoctrinated to think that "right eating" is the same for everybody. That's what ignorant, self-proclaimed slimming gurus seem to think. Well, it's not true. Without being too technical, suffice it to say that we are all a little bit different genetically. I'm not talking about big gene variants but tiny little switches or imperfections among regular genes that we call "single-nucleotide polymorphisms" or SNPs (usually pronounced "snips"!) These SNPs may not be enough for you to grow two heads but might mean, among the many possibilities, that you can't tolerate a certain food very well, even though nobody else has a problem with it.

If you go ahead and eat this food, not knowing it is a problem to you, it will then set up an inflammatory process and cause disturbances in your metabolism that make you feel unwell and maybe retain fluid or gain weight.

Strangely, you could even become addicted to such a food, like a cocaine or heroin addiction. You surely don't need to be told the connection between food addiction and overweight! I'll cover all this in a later section, defining my contribution to nutrition science and healthy eating.

For now, just let it be said that the right diet (for you) is a sensible mix of foods that you tolerate well, enjoy eating, provide adequate nutrition and are satisfying to both taste and visual appeal. Eating a diet of such foods will ensure you are in the best of moods, filled with zest, in tip-top health and steady at your ideal weight. The most important weight-related principle I have learned over the years is that if you are healthy.... really healthy, you *cannot* be overweight.

New Ways To Shed The Pounds

For the sake of clarity, let's state right here at the start, there are only 3 hard-core ways to lose weight. These have been known and understood for more than a century:

- Eat less (counting calories)
- Eat differently (counting carbs, paleo, etc.)
- Exercise more (burn off the excess calories)

Everyone is aware that these take discipline. The perception is that weight loss is hard work. Difficult.

But that's all changing and changing fast. Today's slimmer is more than lucky; there is an abundance of new science that adds many extra tools. Some of them, you will read, don't need much effort. They key is knowing what to do and that's where this book is valuable to you.

It's a fast-fact introduction to things that everyone needs to know about health—but slimmers in particular. For example:

1. Avoidance of manufactured and vitiated foods, with secret addictive formulations
2. Supplements or herbs to modify metabolism
3. Managing "hunger hormones"
4. Controlling systemic inflammation (including knowledge of obesogens)
5. Blood sugar management, including insulin resistance
6. Adjusting your intestinal flora
7. Tune out your "fat" genes
8. Food allergies and addiction
9. Attend to your hormones (especially thyroid hormones)
10. Changing mental patterns

OK, number 2 is a bit simplistic but I just mean the extras you take... supplements, herbs, slimming pills, metabolic enhancers, whatever you want to call them.

Number 6, intestinal flora, will be a puzzling mystery to some but, in fact, could turn out to be the only 100% reliable way to lose weight and not gain it back. It's a complex new development, which I will explain in more detail when we come to it.

You probably know nothing about genes that create obesity problems. But there are quite of few of them! Under this section I include the all-important information about your genomic make up and how you can "tune out" the expression of your obesity genes using carefully chosen supplementation. This will be one of the most important chapters in the book!

Finally, you might think that surgical intervention (bariatric surgery, gastric bypass and liposuction) is a whole different approach but actually it's a subset of eating less (and rather surprisingly, a variant of eating less). I virtually dismiss this approach because it avoids the problems of obesity altogether. Instead of solving a person's self-image defects and nutritional disaster habits, surgical intervention just side steps any learning, change of lifestyle or intelligent reappraisal of one's self-care motives.

I'm not dismissing surgery as only for the weak-minded or foolish, or suggesting that people with low will-power should be punished. I just don't view these surgical interventions as viable health alternatives. But others see it differently and I will share their views and available science with you.

In any case, I have delivered on my promise to cover everything here and later serve up some helpful remarks and details about surgery, to ensure you are fully informed.

Mind And Belief Systems

We all know that weight gain is supposed to be partly a psychological thing: "comfort eating", people's self-image and such-like explanations.

So, what about mind control and hypnosis? Well, I think it's fair to say that counseling methods, hypnosis and such are really aimed at 1 and 2 from the above hard-core list: they get you to eat less, or at least eat differently.

The same could be said for what I call the "disciplinary methods"; Weight Watchers is a good example of this category program, where there is a strong social or peer pressure to conform, to be accountable and eat within suitable limits. That means eating less, inevitably.

But I will allow changes of mental patterns and belief systems to be a valid 6th approach. There is a need for the concept which French Renaissance philosopher Michael de Montaigne called *bien dans sa peau*, or to be "comfortable in one's skin". Being overweight feels negative and uncomfortable. But it is also true that an obsession with slimness and the fashion of supermodels is an undesirable ideal and creates envy and misery for many women. They are not really *bien dans sa peau* either!

These mind-level approaches will be covered in more detail in section 17.

Let's look at each of these fundamental approaches in turn. A lot of what I am going to write is obvious (not all of it) but you would think, to listen to the drivel in TV advertising or the latest glossy magazine ads, that every new plan has come up with something "revolutionary" and "amazing" and "new" when in fact most of it is same-old same-old.

Eat Less!

There is a lot to be said for the oldest belief: to lose weight, just eat less. That's not always the case, as we shall see, but certainly for most Westerners, such as the average Californian consuming thousands of unnecessary, slurping, sugary calories every day and waddling around grossly obese, it is by the far the best and simplest method of losing weight.

That's not to say it's easy, of course, but I'm not here to hold anybody's hand. It's a free country and if someone wants to eat themselves into an early grave, they can; just stay off the aircraft seats near me and don't waste valuable waiting room space in a hospital, looking to repair the damage caused by years of gluttony.

The fact is, we only need a certain amount of calories to get through our busy day and anything over and beyond the basic requirements is redundant. Short-term that doesn't matter but in the long term, over years or decades, such a wasteful lifestyle will eventually catch up with you.

It won't be just obesity, either. The whole process of insulin resistance, blood pressure, heart disease, diabetes and early demise will follow, as night follows day. Remember one simple demographic, if you will: *nobody who makes it to 100 years old is significantly overweight.*

But there is a slight snag to the simplicity of this eat-fewer-calories-and-lose-weight myth. It often doesn't work, except when extreme, and extremes always tend to be more trouble than good.

I said it was simplistic and so it is. It even seems 100% logical. But so many times in my professional working life I have ordered patients to eat more calories (but the right kind) and they have lost weight easily, for the first time in their lives. That's true of the Atkins Diet, for example. By encouraging the consumption of more fats, the appetite is fully satisfied and unnecessary eating vanishes, as food cravings disappear.

Most snacking and nibbling has to do with the fact that the hunger control mechanism or "appestat" (like a thermostat) is not being properly satisfied. The empty yearning continues and so the unlucky individual goes on putting things in the mouth, hoping the feeling will go away. But it doesn't. Then along come fats or oils and suddenly that satisfied "full" feeling manifests and the person no longer feels the need to nibble relentlessly; maybe not for several hours.

Some doctors can't even get their head round such an idea. "It's not possible," they say. "Eating fewer calories is the only way to lose weight."

But consider this: we are biologically designed to store fat when faced with starvation. It's a survival mechanism which goes back to the Stone Age. So if you cut calories and starve, your body thinks there is a hunting crisis—you're all out of woolly mammoths—and goes into fat storage mode!

It's the last thing you want! Your body is fighting your efforts, trying to pile on the fat reserves, while you are trying to do the opposite.

Moreover, going into "starvation mode" adversely affects other aspects of body function too, notably immune function, tissue repair and long-term maintenance.

All in all, then, just cutting calories is a very bad idea.

Eat Differently

Unless you have lived on Planet Zod for years (my favorite joke planet, which is so remote from Earth that nobody there knows anything that's going on down here), you'll have realized that carbohydrates are the real enemy.

What do farmers use to fatten up their livestock and make them gain weight for market? Carbohydrates. What do official government nutritionists insist we all need lots of? Carbohydrates. What have we got as a result? An overweight, unhealthy population. I'm sure you don't need the connection spelled out.

Carbohydrates (most forms) are what we call "empty calories"; they add to the calorie score but do nothing to build healthy, sound minds and bodies. What's more, carbohydrates are unquestionably addictive; when you start eating them you want more... and more and more.

Plus, there is the glycemic index problem. If you indulge in unhealthy levels of carbohydrate intake, you will upset your body's glucose control mechanisms. This will lead to obesity, diabetes, hypertension, heart disease and the whole chronic cardiac early-death cycle; it rejoices in the name of metabolic syndrome or just "diabesity".

The fact is that you often need only limit carbohydrates in your diet to have comfortable and dramatic weight loss.

Heck, you can eat as much as you want of anything that doesn't have carbs in it! Effectively that means all meat, all fish, all fowl, almost all vegetables and almost all fruits. What could be better?

You can clear a plate of sirloin, broccoli, peas and artichoke fries for a count of virtually zero! If you are still hungry, cook and eat the same meal all over again! No score! That's my kind of dieting.

What's more, Nature loves this program. It's like being hunter-gatherers: lots of protein (flesh), to show we have been successful in our hunting!

Low carb dieting is much easier than low calorie dieting. In the latter everything that passes your lips is added to the overall score. It can be miserable, counting calories. You feel such a failure when you get really hungry and find you have to eat something because you are feeling so faint you'll fall over. That happens with low calorie diets but it means you cheated! Then the whole guilt thing starts... Remember poor old Bridget Jones (*Bridget Jones Diary* movie, starring Renée Zellweger, 2001)!

With low carb eating when you feel faint, just knock back a handful of cashews and (if you must) a smoothie made of carrots, avocado, coconut water and berries. Yum! Roll up a slice of ham and nibble, like a candy bar. Weight loss continues uninterrupted. Hunger is not a problem.

Other Ways Of Eating Differently

There are many ways to follow the eating differently path. The Atkins Diet and The Paleo-Diet, are both tested and proven methods that come up trumps time and time again, despite efforts to discredit them that seem to go on and on relentlessly.

There are absurd extremes, which I will not even consider, like the "Cabbage Soup Diet". It might as well be called the "Belsen Diet" because it's just about as healthy as the swill served in a concentration camp.

Due to the ridiculous food pyramid foisted on us by idiot government scientists back in the 1970s, supposed correct eating appears to include a lot of carbohydrate. So avoiding the follies of the food pyramid may make most plans seem "low carbohydrate" in character. Really this is not so. Nature's own diet we should follow (the hunter-gatherer pattern) defines proper carbohydrate levels that are far lower than what we have become used to.

In fact the low-carbohydrate plan has a long history and goes back way earlier than these modern takes. The first successful description of such a diet was that published by William Banting (1796 - 1878). The method even became known for a time as "Banting", after its founder.

In 1967, Irwin Stillman published *The Doctor's Quick Weight Loss Diet*. The "Stillman Diet" is a high-protein, low-carbohydrate and low-fat diet. It is regarded as one of the first low-carbohydrate diets to become popular in the United States.

There is nothing new in these plans and the fact they are still in circulation means one thing: the low-carb method works and works well.

And by the way, ignore all those fake studies, which purport to show eating meat is bad for you. I have yet to see such a study! The ones that are claimed to show meat and saturated fats are bad always screw up the data by including consumption of obese, unhealthy fatty animals (up to 30% fat in their meats), or manufactured meat filth (processed meat, junk-burgers, pink slime, mechanically recovered meats, spam, etc.) These agri-business nightmare products are NOT red meat!

Pure red meat, on its own (and in moderation), is what we are supposed to eat. You know what? It's very healthy to eat meat from animals which are kept on free-range pastures and fed natural organic foods. Among other benefits, this grass-fed beef contains the highest known levels of healthy omega-3 fatty acids. I'll deal with the issue of vegetarianism and its supposed merits later.

My own contribution will be to make sure that you understand fully why the so-called hunter-gatherer diet is natural to humans and why it is Nature-designed to provide health for a slim, active, mobile species like us. Why fight Nature? She knows what she is doing.

Kellogg's, Kraft, Nestlé, PepsiCo, McDonald's and all the other propagandists are there to make money, not make you healthy.

Exercise More

We all know that if you want to lose weight, you work out in the gym, right? Thrash through a good cardio program two or three times a week, get lathered in sweat, and just watch those pounds fall off!

Wrong. Cardio is not a good option, actually! In fact has been proven a poor choice for weight loss; interval training is better. But exercise is not a good way to lose weight, despite many other obvious health benefits.

There are plenty of reasons to exercise, including cardiac efficiency and beating aging. I'm all for it, though in moderation; and people are often shocked when they learn that hard exercise can be very damaging to the body and will actually shorten your life. More is definitely NOT better!

A 2012 study in the *European Heart Journal* found that long-term endurance athletes suffer from diminished function of the right ventricle of the heart and increased cardiac enzymes (markers for heart injury) after endurance racing, which may activate platelet formation and clotting. Twelve percent of the athletes had detectable scar tissue on their heart muscle one week post-race. [1]

In any case, as a path to weight loss, exercise is way too much hard work! I mean, if you play an hour of strenuous tennis, swimming or pushing weights in the gym, you'll burn maybe 600 - 700 calories.

That's roughly equivalent to one cup of sugar. I have always thought it's easier to give up the sugar! Of course, I did give up sugar many years ago. But consider that a half cup (about 2 oz.) of Alfredo pasta sauce can be 500 calories, or that a quarter pound cheeseburger and fries needs about 2 hours of jogging or fast walking to work it off, and you'll see that carefully choosing what you eat can produce far more effective weight control than hours spent working out every week.

Let's put this another way:

According to the Mayo Clinic website, because 3,500 calories equals about 1 pound (0.45 kilogram) of fat, you need to burn 3,500 calories more than you take in to lose 1 pound. So if you cut 500 calories from your diet each day, you'd lose about 1 pound a week (500 calories x 7 days = 3,500 calories).

The equivalent in exercise is one hour of hard sweat every single day. No question, then, that eating differently is the easier option than toil.

It's worth noting however, that while diet has a stronger effect on weight loss than physical activity does, once you've lost the weight, physical exercise has a measurable role to play in maintaining weight loss in the long term. I'll come back to this point at the end, in the section on maintenance of ideal weight.

Of course, as I said, there are other very good reasons to exercise. You need to be active. You need to stay supple and flexible. With plenty of physical activity we feel alert, lively, vigorous, focused and, as a matter of fact, less likely to overeat.

A 2016 study even showed that physical exercise counters most of the negative health effects of alcohol.[2]

For most healthy adults, the US Department of Health and Human Services recommends these exercise guidelines:

<u>Aerobic activity</u>. Get at least 150 minutes a week of moderate aerobic activity or 75 minutes a week of vigorous aerobic activity. However, to effectively lose or maintain weight, some people may need up to 300 minutes a week of moderate physical activity. You also can do a combination of moderate and vigorous activity. The guidelines suggest that you spread out this exercise during the course of a week, and sessions of activity should be at least 10 minutes in duration.

<u>Strength training</u>. Do strength training exercises at least twice a week. No specific amount of time for each strength training session is included in the guidelines.

Moderate aerobic exercise includes such activities as brisk walking, swimming and mowing the lawn. Vigorous aerobic exercise includes such activities as running and aerobic dancing.

Strength training can include use of weight machines, or activities such as rock climbing or heavy gardening.

<u>Dance Exercizing</u>: don't feel that "working out" or jogging are the only useful exercises. The success of dance routines, such as Jazzercise (www.jazzercise.com) and Zumba Fitness (www. zumbafitness. com) means you can have fun, get high on rhythm and lose weight.

You should also consider Dr. Al Sear's P.A.C.E. program (though how you can patent exercises is beyond me).

Short Walk Kills Cravings

Where exercise can really score is that it helps reduce appetite by knocking out cravings; nothing to do with burning off calories. Here's an interesting confirmatory study of that.

Researchers at Exeter University (UK) studied a group of 78 people who were regular chocolate eaters but had gone two days without eating chocolate. They were divided into four groups.

Two groups took a brisk 15-minute walk on a treadmill and then were given either an easy, low- stress task or a more difficult, high-stress task to complete at a desk. The two other groups had a rest instead of walking before being given either the easy or difficult task.

Now this is interesting: all the participants had a bowl of chocolate on their desks while they worked on their tasks! What do you think happened?

On average, those who exercised before doing the task ate half the amount of chocolate as those who rested before the task—15 grams versus 28 grams. Fifteen grams is equivalent to a small, "fun-size" chocolate bar.

It didn't make a difference whether the individuals were engaged in a difficult or easy task, which suggests that stress does not influence the cravings for sweet snacks, the University of Exeter researchers pointed out in the report published online in the journal *Appetite*.

What made the difference was exercise.

We all know that snacking at work on high-calorie foods, like chocolate, can become a mindless habit and will certainly lead to weight gain over time. We justify it by telling ourselves that these snacks give us an energy boost, or help us overcome the boredom. Maybe that's so.

But you have at least one tool to beat the cravings. This study shows that by taking a short walk, you can regulate your intake, reducing it by almost half.[3]

Herbal Supplements

The idea of taking herbs to either curb the appetite (eat less without feeling hungry) or alter metabolism (same intake, but lose weight) has enormous appeal to the slimmer with discipline problems or emotionally-driven eating.

Taking a supplement and losing weight "quickly and easily" as the TV ads claim, has always attracted the overweight majority. But it's a hollow message, trust me.

First: all the ads are a fraud. When you read the fine print, or listen to the fast-gab, they say eat less, exercise regularly and take our stuff and you will lose weight. In almost every case, if you just eat less and exercise regularly, as they recommend, you'll lose weight anyway! You don't need to buy their formula!

Secondly, this sort of approach lacks the value of learning about the mechanisms of weight control so that you can become self-regulating. Believe it or not, it is possible to learn how to get rid of food cravings, addictions and indulgent desires by learning how they come about and how to switch them off. Surely that's more valuable than just popping a pill or powder?

Most of the compounds lack good science. They rely heavily on testimonials, meaning somebody wants to boast they lost 50 – 100 lbs. and the manufacturers claim it was entirely due to their formula. This blatant lack of real science should put you on your guard.

Beware also of deliberately fake science, designed to gull the public, like that which backs up the "Sprinkles" formula (biggest hoax in the market).

Having said that, there are some things worth considering. Data for conjugated linoleic acid (CLA), *Garcinia cambogia* (hydroxycitric acid), chitosan, pyruvate, *Irvingia gabonensis*, chia seeds and camu camu show they appear to be effective in weight loss via fat modifying mechanisms; that's according to a study published recently in the Journal Of Obesity. [4]

However, the data on the use of these products is limited, the article said, and advised caution.

I would add one or two successful compounds that this study did not take into account and which definitely have health value, over and above the question of weight control. See section 10 for listings of useful weight loss supplements. Just don't rely entirely on them, OK?

As an aside, if you are looking for the maximum and fastest benefit with any herbal preparation, consider taking it in liquid form rather than pill form (Hoodia, for example). When you use an extract in liquid form it absorbs into the body 95 percent faster than pills. Pills have to break down and for people who really have trouble containing their hunger, they may eat until the pills start working. So, if you are one of those people who have a hard time getting disciplined then try taking the liquid form. You may see a big difference.

Adjusting Your Intestinal Flora

Probably the biggest secret of all to weight control is this one. In fact the truth is slowly coming around to the fact that this is the number one crucial aspect of obesity that has been hidden from us till recently. Science is now pushing out new boundaries.

The type of micro-organisms which share your intestinal tract are not just passengers; far from it. They are an integral part of our bigger, "biological self" and can exert enormous influence for good or bad.

These microbes carry a vast array of DNA material which, it has been discovered, can actually influence the performance of human cells. This is a shocking surprise: you would expect that only human genes could influence the human body.

Now we have grasped this important fact, you will readily see that the type of microbes we carry around with us will have great influence on our health. There can be "good" and "bad" intestinal flora; those which help us and those which cause issues.

Not surprisingly then, it has been discovered that our bowel flora influences our tendency to gain weight considerably. In fact, as I said, it could be the number one influence! I'll walk you through this in a later section.

The Fatso Gene, The Atkins Gene and Others

The FTO gene (nicknamed the "Fatso" gene) is not the only gene that carries the tendency to be overweight. I have listed several others for you, such as fat absorption gene 2 (FAB2), PPARγ (lipid metabolism) and two "fat burning" genes. ADRβ2 is associated with carbohydrate cravings, which make weight control extremely difficult.

And, yes, there is a gene which mimics the Atkins diet: it's nicknamed the Atkins gene. You'll find out why later!

This is unavoidable material and is a huge missing slice of the dieting market. I will rectify that gap. I will be telling the reader where and how to get a reliable gene profile and how to work to tone down harmful combinations and tune up the helpful variants (this is called epigenetics). It's not just supplements: vitamin D quells inflammation for example and the "right" type of exercise for a particular gene variant is critical too.

So-called vitamin D receptors need to be understood. Vitamin D regulates at least 900 other genes, controlling inflammation and obesity.

Changing Mental Patterns

Only a fool today would doubt the influence of mental states on all aspects of health. Open any woman's magazine on a regular basis and soon you will see the connection drawn between being overweight and deep personal issues, such as self-image, sexuality and contentment.

Everyone understands the label "comfort food" for mindless eating when you are upset and in emotional turmoil.

Plus there is no question that stress of all kinds will add to weight problems. Chronic stress (the usual kind today) leads to excess secretions of the main "stress hormone" cortisol. That in turn has many potentially dangerous side effects, such as thinning of the bones, stomach damage, water retention, skin conditions and hypertension, not to mention memory loss, depression and actual brain damage.

But one other side effect is beyond question: cortisol can cause weight gain. Not only that but, unfortunately, it has the characteristic pattern of fat deposit in the belly area, just where we don't want it. Belly fat, as you will read later, is especially dangerous to health, being associated with heart disease and stroke.

Moreover, a recent meta-analysis study has drawn a strong association between stress and inflammatory cytokines, which can be released from belly fat.[5]

What I am saying here is that stress can lead to weight gain, not just via mindless eating, but through hidden chemical signaling influences.

Unless you deal with the stress, these hidden cytokine effects will remain beyond your control and prevent you losing weight as you would wish. So relieving stress and strain could be a very important slimming intervention! Learn more about controlling stress in section 17.

In fact some people see this as the only thing you need to do to lose weight: clean up your emotional act and you'll have no trouble sticking to a diet plan; the pounds will tumble off.

Well, it isn't that simple. You will find shocking revelations in this volume, such as the fact that two different people can eat the same food exactly, taking corresponding degrees of exercise, and yet one lose weight and the other not. In such cases, thyroid status, for example, can have a profound influence. So can hidden chemicals, deliberately added to our foods.

Is all this making sense? Don't you find this more valuable and more appealing than dumb slimming books that just say eat less calories or count your carbs?

Other Vitally Significant Factors That Control Weight

You will read about so-called "hunger hormones", chemical messengers that, when working properly, act to tell you that you are hungry and need to eat, or that you have eaten sufficient and should stop!

We know that the thyroid gland secretes a number of hormones, levels of which work as our biological accelerator pedal, speeding up or slowing down metabolism. Obviously if our internal "engine" runs faster, we burn fuel faster and lose weight easily. Conversely, if we are sluggish, we have trouble losing weight. This is the condition of low thyroid function and it plagues probably the majority of women; certainly very many individuals have undiagnosed thyroid dysfunction and it plays havoc with health and weight.

There are other hormones too which directly influence your fat levels and hence weight.

Environmental pollution may surprise the reader as a newly emerged and understood factor influencing our fat levels. We now have the concept of *obesogens* (chemicals which generate obesity), a term coined by Professor Bruce Blumberg at the University of California, Irvine. Any savvy woman knows that estrogen causes weight gain and water retention (not to mention changes in mood). Well, we now have uncontrolled estrogenic-mimicking substances (such as bisphenol-A) loose in our environment—sufficient to cause faulty growth in males and lowered sperms counts—and sufficient to give rise to all the unpleasant side effects of unwanted estrogen.

There are a number of other surprising factors that influence weight, such as sleep patterns, general inflammation, parasites and food allergies, which you will read about in upcoming chapters.

Diets Reviewed

With all that in mind, the later part of the book is given over to reviewing quite a number of the major and fashionable approaches to weight loss that are around. I've even included the no-no diets and suggested to you why these are not a good approach to use.

I've tried to give them a personal rating but this must, of necessity, remain an opinion. For example I give the low carb method 5 stars and the low calorie method 2 stars. Both work but the low carb method is easier and more enjoyable than counting calories. The latter means that anything whatsoever you eat will count to your daily score. So breaking it and taking a nibble because you feel desperate means you spoil your score and then feel guilty and miserable; all bad stuff.

But with the low carb approach, you can snack on nuts, vegetables, cold meats or tinned fish (to name just a few examples), without any score whatever! You can't drink wine on a low calorie diet: one gram of alcohol has almost as many calories as fats (7 calories in alcohol, to 9 calories in fat). Whereas a glass of wine is zero on the carb counting system (one glass a day limit when you are trying to slim).

I'll go into all this in detail, when we get to the appropriate comparisons.

FINALLY, I'll venture to offer and explain what is probably the best, most scientific, most natural and actually the fastest way to lose weight and feel good, without experiencing hunger. Yes, there is such a plan and I'll share it with you in full, before the end! Stay with me!

OK, enough preamble. Let's get started...

PART 1. THE BASICS

SECTION 2. BEGINNER'S STUFF: THE BASICS CONCEPTS YOU NEED TO KNOW

Hunger: Is There More Than One Kind?

There are many stimuli for eating and just talking about "hunger" is vague and inadequate. For sure, hunger isn't always lack of nourishment. Even well fed or obese individuals can feel hungry, though this isn't exactly natural.

The impulse to eat can come from food addictions, as we shall see; from the secretion of hormones that regulate the feelings of hunger and feeling "full"; it can come simply from habit or the clock ("Now it's lunchtime"); the desire to initiate a meal can come from a pleasant anticipation of flavors and appearance of mouth-watering recipes (watching TV cookery shows can initiate the desire to eat, though that's not hunger, of course). Eating can be a strong social event, meaning we want to sit down to a meal for companionship with people we like or love and in this situation the food is merely an excuse for a friendly gathering, rather than hunger or the desire to eat. And then there is the matter of comfort eating: indulging in food as a solution to emotional distress or tension.

These are the many faces of hunger or perhaps we can say "hungers", plural. All the ones I have detailed above have little to do with lack of nourishment, you will agree.

What we know is that humans eat episodically, meaning not all the time, like grazing animals do. With meals, people usually eat until they are comfortably full, after which they do not eat for a certain time (not hungry).

Immediately after a meal, there is a low drive to eat. This drive builds up again until the moment of the next eating episode.

Instead of this vague word hunger, we'll take our cue from papers published by J Hartnell and J Blundell and cited in the *American Journal of Clinical Nutrition* in 2004. These two authors defined the terms **satiation**, solving your hunger, meaning getting to the point of satisfaction with sufficient food—and **satiety**, not needing to eat, the feeling before hunger strikes. Both of these terms are obviously related to the word satisfaction.

This is made more complicated by the fact that people do not always eat when they are hungry, and they do not always refrain from eating when satiated.

Satiation is influenced by how much we eat but the type of food is also crucial and it is far from a simple accounting process or quantification. Satiety tells us how satisfying and valuable recent meals have been, regulating whether or not we feel hungry quite soon after food or whether we can go for hours without more intake. Satiation is an indicator of meal termination; satiety is an indicator of meal initiation (when satiety levels drop).

There can be other sensory factors that signal "enough food" (tight belt sensation, for example), or metabolic factors (such as changes in blood sugar levels). Most peoples' regulation of eating is controlled by a mixture of sensory modalities.

Then there are hunger hormones. We all know that scientists like something to measure. So can we turn satiety and satiation into some numbers? There seem to be three viable biomarkers, which correlate instructively with the sensation of hunger. These are blood insulin levels, leptin and ghrelin.

We'll look at these in more detail when the time comes. Other possible markers that are being looked at are blood concentrations of cholecystokinin and glucagon-like peptide 1 (GLP-1) but these are too technical for our needs in this volume.

Why It Really Is Bad To Eat Quickly

Then let's introduce another complication: **saturation**, as it is called. This is the phenomenon in which food molecules are given time to permeate the body, so that the control mechanisms of the "appestat" (like a thermostat) are triggered. Without this phenomenon, the body wouldn't really know its feeding intake or nutritional status, so it's an important concept.

What it boils down to is this: fast eaters get bad results because they beat their appestat and are already consuming more than they need, before the signals kick in that say, "I have eaten enough."

Saturation appears to be related to the time that it takes the senses to perceive the product. For this reason, calories in liquid form impact quicker than eating the food in a solid form. Soup, however, saturates because it is eaten slowly with a spoon. So liquid foods will tend to be overeaten, whereas slow chewy ones won't.

This is why we advize eating slowly (page 195). It's even been suggested that people who want to lose weight should try eating with chopsticks!

Then there is the matter of choices, which has little to do with quantification. The reasons we choose the foods we do come from a variety of input stimuli but these choices are definitely a part of the motivation to eat. The preparation, smell, appearance and taste of food all impact on the question of food choices, yet it seems to me that scientists put far too little emphasis on this matter which, to epicurians like me, could be the most powerful motivation to eat.

All of this makes it difficult to investigate eating qualitatively (WHAT a person eats, as opposed to how much). Even so, questionnaires do have some value in making determinations. Most investigators who use rating scales to assess appetite use the terminology developed by Rogers and Blundell at the end of the 1970s:

- hunger
- desire to eat
- prospective consumption
- fullness

These terms relate to slightly different aspects of the motivation to eat. Prospective consumption (or "How much can you eat?") seems to be an easier and more concrete question than vague questions about hunger. "Hunger" may refer to the appetite for a meal, whereas "desire to eat" may refer to a milder, pleasant feeling of appetite for a snack. "Fullness" refers to a satisfied sensation in the stomach.

"Appetite" as such can be inferred, if not directly measured, by recording actual food intake; that is, the amount of food eaten within a certain context can be considered as a measure of appetite. But the degree to which actual food intake reflects appetite is debatable.

However, it is generally agreed that direct measurement of intake is preferable to self-assessment by individuals, who tend to notoriously over or under-estimate what they have eaten (hence the food diary tool referred to later in this section). [1]

Keeping Track Of Your Slimming Progress

Let's now look at the most basic of basics: measuring progress in weight loss. You might think that's easy: get a set of decent bathroom scales and step on them. It's not so simple.

We are talking here about weight loss, so of course you want to measure weight and look for progress. But it isn't the only issue.

For example, you may have heard that athletes can sometimes gain weight when they work out; muscle weighs more than fat, so if you trim the fat, work out and pile on muscle, you might end up weighing rather more!

Also, typical bathroom scales are not always reliable. You need to weigh yourself on the same scales every time, because they vary so much.

As metal springs age they go stiffer. What does that mean? They stretch more reluctantly and won't let the needle on the dial get right around to your true weight. In other words they lie and tell you that you are lighter than you really are. You probably weigh more than you think you do.

Get a proper weight on a balance arm scale—you know, the kind where you are balanced against weights slid along a beam. These are accurate to within 0.5% or less. You can get a true weight like this at your doctor's office; make sure they have the right scales—the nurse will probably do it for you for no cost. Then check that against your bathroom scales on the same day and if the difference is more than 5- 6 lbs, junk the spring scales.

Junk them anyway after about 2 years max.

How Often Should You Weigh Yourself?

There is some controversy about how often to step on the scales. Some schools say do it daily; keep track; know what's going on. Others think it's being less neurotic to weigh yourself once a week... or even less. Being over-sensitive to your weight issues may lead to the build-up of an eating disorder.

Those who think you should weigh yourself daily point to the fact that it keeps weight control uppermost in your mind. It invites discipline. Also, you will soon learn to relate certain eating behaviors with their effect on your progress. It's depressing to have a blow out and realize that you have gained back 4 hard-won pounds! But that's better than fooling yourself and the shock and upset may make you all the more determined.

Those who advocate weighing yourself less often point out that daily fluctuations are very natural, unavoidable and don't mean very much. What appears to be a temporary blip may not signal a problem and should not cause you to re-evaluate your whole program and maybe change for something else.

Choose what works best for you, psychologically.

But one important fact everyone is agreed on, whether it's daily, weekly or monthly: weigh yourself at the same time of day each time. Otherwise you are not comparing like with like. Incredibly, a person's weight may vary by several pounds during the course of a single day. I'm talking up to five pounds variation (depending on your starting weight), due to eating, drinking and sweating from activity.

So, to avoid unnecessary upset and confusion, decide to weigh yourself first thing in the morning, nude and before you eat or drink anything.

Measuring Your Fat Load

A CT scan or MRI is the only precise way to see where fat is stored. But there are quick calculations that can show how you might be storing your fat.

One of the simplest checks you can make, which most experts agree indicates if you may have unsafe levels of visceral fat, is to measure your waist circumference. If it's over 35 inches for a woman and over 40 inches for a man, that's a red alert.

Here are instructions on measuring your waist accurately from the National Heart Lung and Blood Institute:

1. Stand up. Exhale before you measure - do not suck in your breath.
2. Wrap the tape measure around your middle. It should go across your navel.
3. Make sure bottom of the tape measure is just above your hip bones. It does not go higher up, even if you're narrower there.

Body Mass Index (BMI) was a fashionable obesity measure for a time. Trouble is, a superb mountain-of-muscle athlete like basketball player Michael Jordan would be technically obese, using this measure. That's absurd.

What BMI is doing is to compare your weight to your size, using a supposed surface area measurement. It goes back a surprisingly long time; originally known as the Quetelet index, it was devised around 1840 by the Belgian polymath Adolphe Quetelet (1796–1874) during the course of developing his "social physics".

Body mass index is defined as the individual's body mass divided by the square of their height. The formulae universally used in medicine produces a unit of measure of kg/m2.

BMI = mass in kg/ height in metres^2

If you want to work in pounds and inches (US and UK):

BMI = mass in lbs/ height in inches x 703

To work from stones and pounds first multiply the stone by 14 then add the pounds to give the whole mass in pounds; to work from feet and inches first multiply the feet by 12 then add the inches to give the whole height in inches.

BMI can also be quickly determined using a BMI chart, which displays BMI as a function of weight (horizontal axis) and height (vertical axis) using contour lines for different values of BMI or colors for different BMI categories.

But you don't have to do any math or use a chart; you can find BMI calculators all over the Internet. The best advice however is to forget about them.

What's The Measurement That Really Matters?

What's the most important measure for healthy weight? Waist-to-hip ratio. It has been shown scientifically that this measurement relates more accurately to health problems than the now-discredited BMI.

Simply put, excess fat in the abdominal region (belly fat) poses a greater health risk than excess fat in the hips and thighs and is associated with a significantly higher risk of high blood pressure, diabetes, early onset of heart disease, and certain types of cancers (American Dietetic Association). See section 3 for a fuller explanation of the dangers of belly fat.

This newer measurement is potentially more telling than simply weighing yourself, as body composition and fat distribution is a more meaningful indicator of health outcomes.

To determine your own WTH ratio measure yourself round the widest part of your abdomen (let it out, no cheating!) Then do the same round your hips. Men should be 1:1 maximum (waist same as hips). Women should be 0.85 (waist at least 1- 2 inches less than the hips).

And gals, remember waist-to-hip is what attracts guys the most!

Pears, Apples and Scrawny

It's not just how much fat. Having a "pear shape," with fatter hips and thighs, is considered safer than the "apple shape," which describes a wider waistline. This is why your waist-to-hip ratio is more valuable as a health monitor than just BMI, which makes no allowance for *where* your fat is stored.

Typically, if you are at a healthy weight, you'll have healthy levels of visceral fat, as well. But genes can predispose a person to being thin and still having a disproportionate amount of visceral fat, which is dangerous.

And in case you are wondering: being thin in every dimension is bad too. Skinny isn't good. People who are underweight do not live as long as those who are slightly overweight. Normal or correct weight is best. But to be a bit overweight is healthier than being skinny. This might seem paradoxical. But Nature always has a different point of view from arrogant, cocky scientists!

A Scandinavian study (Denmark) indicates that even thighs can be measured to give a prediction of longevity and that thin thighs are bad. Supermodels beware! If you don't die of a drugs overdose, you will probably die young anyway! Not that fat thighs are good. But thin thighs are definitely a risk factor. After studying nearly 3,000 men and women for over 12 years, researchers concluded that a thigh circumference of 24 inches (around 60 centimeters) is ideal.

The report, by researchers at Copenhagen University Hospital, was published in the Sept. 4, 2009 issue of the *British Medical Journal.* This new measurement is an addition to using BMI (body-mass index).

It seems odd as to why a thin thigh may predict heart disease. However, it could represent that fat and muscle is not being deposited in the right place where it is needed, and certainly we know that fat in wrong places, such as skeletal muscle and liver and pancreas, is associated with diabetes and may increase mortality.

So the problem here may not be with the thin thighs, but where else the bulk is going.[2]

Percentage Body Fat

Better than measuring your weight, is to keep track of percentage body fat. Fat, remember, is lighter than muscle and sinew. So if you work out vigorously and become hardened and muscular, you could end up weighing more, yet be in healthier shape.

The real worry, as you will later learn, is the quantity of visceral fat you are carrying around. That's the fat packed around your heart, gut, spleen and kidneys (like suet!) It's very unhealthy, highly inflammatory and leads directly to cardiovascular trouble (heart attack, stroke, early death). Get rid of it! That's what these pages are about.

However, you need to measure how much is there. Not easy; you can't just fling a tape measure round it! So we have to estimate the quantity electronically. You can get health and obesity monitoring systems, like the Omron scale, which will give you a read out of weight, BMI (estimate), total body fat (a percentage), visceral fat (as a percentage) and muscle bulk as a percentage of your total weight.

It works because muscle, bone and fat have different electrical impedances and the machines are cleverly programmed to figure it all out.

You stand on a scale with electrode pads that make contact with the soles of your feet and hold (two-handed) a set of electrodes and the scale does the rest. You need to input your age, height and gender, of course (women are allowed a different percentage of body fat for men). The important thing is not so much the absolute values, as keeping track of change over time (relative improvement).

For fit men, we are looking for a percentage body fat of less than 20%; for women, that should be 25% or less but these targets depend a lot on age, so you will need tables (supplied with the Omron scale).

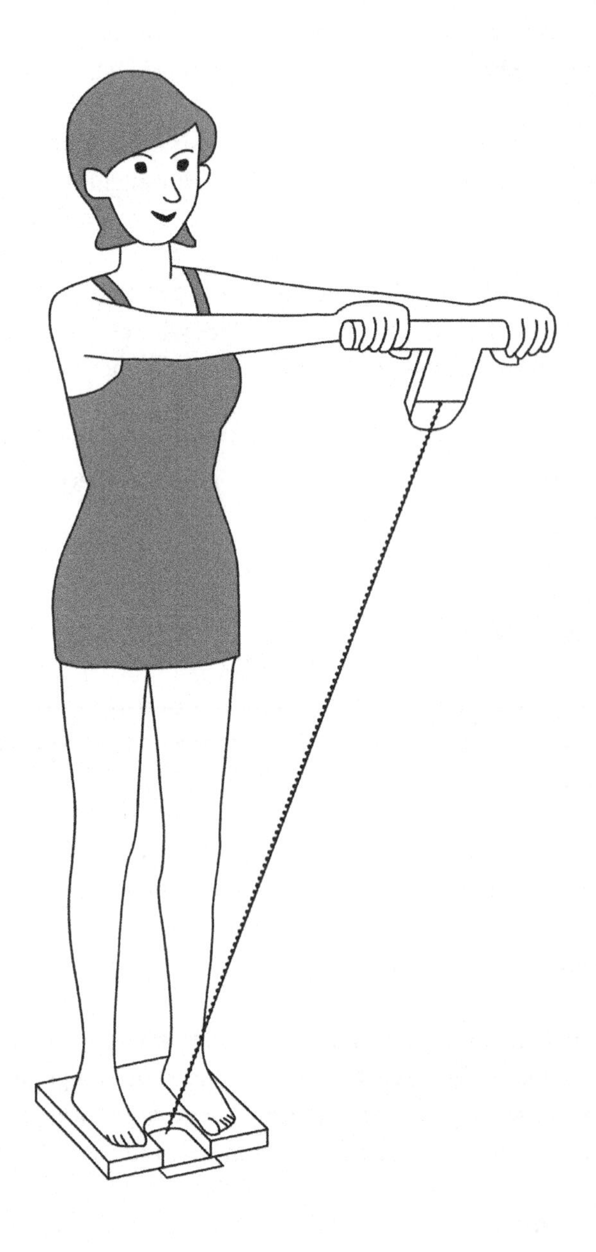

Calipers

One final measurement may be useful and that's measuring subcutaneous fat using calipers. It's sometimes known as the skin-fold method or "pinch test".

You are measuring something different to the dreaded "belly fat". Calipers detect subcutaneous body fat in specific areas; meaning the fat that lies just under the skin. Sports men and women, gym enthusiasts and body-builders love it. But it has little meaning in terms of overall health.

The main drawback of the skin-fold method is that you can't do it accurately on yourself. That's because the best test areas (abdomen and thighs) are not easy to reach, without distorting them by bending over.

But it's also complicated: you take several measurements and average them.

Then you have a choice of over 100 equations to use, for calculating the "true" body fat percentage! Each equation relates to different populations of people with different characteristics. Young people for example, store about one half of their body fat under the skin. As we age a greater proportion of our body fat is stored internally.

Gender, fitness level, race and the amount of total body fat a person has, also make a difference. So it's probably best left the enthusiasts who want to pursue this as a measure of success and fitness.

How accurate is the caliper method?

An article published in the *Journal of the American Dietetic Association* showed a considerable correlation between the skin-fold method and computed tomography (CAT scan) measurements, making it a clinically useful and pretty accurate measurement. [3]

But that assumes you are using high quality calipers, like in a scientific study. So forget the $10 cheap junk. You need to invest in good skin-fold calipers that can cost several hundred dollars. It may be worth it, if you are taking yourself very seriously!

The top 5 skin-fold calipers, recommended by Phil at the Sports Fitness Advisor website are:

Harpenden Skinfold Caliper

The Harpenden is the most accurate skinfold caliper made. It has been the standard research caliper for many years. Virtually all the data and equations relating skinfold thickness to body fat are based on studies done with the Harpenden.

Lafayette Skinfold Caliper

The Lafayette Skinfold Caliper is one of the most accurate and durable calipers available today. It was designed with the assistance of Dr. Andrew Jackson, co- author of the widely used Jackson and Pollock skinfold formulas.

Lange Caliper

This is the best-selling of the higher priced body fat calipers. It has been manufactured since 1962 and is widely used in schools, colleges and fitness centers. The Lange is one of the lower cost professional calipers.

Accu-Measure Body Fat Calipers

At the moment these are the only body fat calipers that reliably let you test yourself. They are extremely simple to use and a recent study has shown very positive results for accuracy. Recommended in Body-for-LIFE and endorsed by the World Natural Bodybuilding Federation.

Slim Guide Skinfold Caliper

Much lower priced than any of the above body fat calipers yet will produce results that are almost as accurate. This is the only low cost caliper accurate enough to be used for professional measurements and is the most widely used professional caliper in the world.

Keep A Food Diary

If you want to lose weight, you probably need to eat less - and if you want to eat less, it helps to write down what you are doing. This is an important tracking tool.

When researchers studied the eating behaviors of female dieters they found that the most important tool linked to successful weight loss was a pen and notebook. It's called a "food diary" or food journal.

Women who kept food journals and consistently wrote down the foods they ate lost more weight than women who didn't.

What's more, researchers found that skipping meals and eating out frequently, especially at lunch, led to less weight loss. That's according to a study which appeared in the latest issue of the Journal of the Academy of Nutrition and Dietetics.

Over the course of a year, the women followed a restricted-calorie diet with the goal of achieving a 10% reduction in weight in six months. Half the women were put on an exercise program and the other half were not. All the participants were asked to record the foods they ate daily in seven-day diaries provided weekly by dietician counselors.

At the end of the year, both the diet-alone and diet-and-exercise groups had lost an average of 10% of their starting weight. But... here's the kicker: women who consistently filled out a food journal lost about 6 pounds more than those who didn't.

Those who skipped meals lost an average of 8 fewer pounds than those who didn't.

Women who ate in restaurants at lunch at least once a week lost an average of 5 pounds less than those who ate out less.

This isn't a one-off study, either: a 2008 study found that dieters who kept food diaries at least six days a week lost twice as much weight as those who kept the journals one day a week or less.

Incidentally, it's best to write down the foods you eat as soon as you eat them, rather than waiting until the end of the day. [4]

Why should keeping a food journal help? Seems straightforward: it helps to prevent mindless eating.

Weight Loss Smartphone Apps

One more aid or tool that you might consider, which has many of the positive properties of a food diary, is a smartphone app. There are a number available to help you, some free and some you have to pay a modest sum for. I have put notes about these into appendix 1.

OK, next up is the first of my "Quick and Simple Diets"!

Quick and Simple Diet #1. Cut up your food!

This is one of a series of quick-fix changes you can make that will give you nearly instant results, while you continue to read and learn the real "Science Of Slimming".

Cut up your food!

Fact: we feel full faster, and eat less later, when our food is served in small pieces.

Cut up your food and chew it properly, every Mum worth her salt knows that.

But it seems eating smaller mouthfuls is another way to lose weight. It works in both college students and lab rats, according to a study by Devina Wadhera and her colleagues at Arizona State University.

The researchers first tried this on lab rats. The animals were trained to run through a maze. Then the animals were offered a reward for running quickly through the maze. For 20 rats, the reward was a single chunk of food. For another 20 rats, the reward was 30 small pieces of food weighing the same as the large piece offered to the other rats.

After 12 trips through the maze, the result was clear. Rats preferred—and worked harder for—the same amount of food served in smaller pieces.

Okay, it's easy to fool a rat. But what about college students? (even easier, some might say!)

Wadhera's team split 301 male and female students into two groups. One was offered a whole bagel covered with cream cheese. The other group was offered the same kind of bagel, cut into four pieces and covered with the same amount of cream cheese.

The group that got the whole bagel ate a little more of it than those who got the cut-up bagel. But the real difference came 20 minutes later, when all of the students were offered a free meal.

Those who'd eaten the cut-up bagel—even though they'd eaten a little less—ate less of the free meal.

Wow, if it gets college kids to refuse free food, it really must work!

The study was presented at the annual meeting of the Society for the Study of Ingestive Behavior, held in Zurich, Switzerland. [5]

My 21 Hottest Weight Loss Tips

OK, for those in a hurry to get some visible results, take a look at these 20 key points and get acting on them. You could see benefits within just a few days!

1. Eat Smaller Portions

OK, it seems obvious. But think it through:

If you are overweight but stable—even 50 lbs overweight or more, but you are not continuing to gain—you only need to eat a very little less to start to lose. A 10% reduction in what you eat, which would hardly be a misery, should get you going on a long, slow weight loss process. Of course this doesn't apply if you are still overdoing things and continuing to gain weekly; only if your weight is steady.

If you eat out, choose well and eat only half; ask for the rest to be boxed and take it home for the next day (great economy, by the way).

2. Try To Be Less Interested In Food

If you just live for food and can't wait for your next gourmet thrill, you'll have trouble sticking to any diet. A good meal, with good food and great company is one of life's wonderful moments. But to lose weight, you need to get very bored with what you eat! Get to the state where you couldn't care less what's for lunch or dinner! Celebrate the lack of interest, instead of angst over it! But you can also get to like the "boring" foods—cabbage or sprouts can be much more lively if you cook them in a little chicken stock, with some bacon chunks to add flavor!

3. Don't Eat "By The Clock"

This is a big mistake people get into; it becomes a negative life habit. You know, it's the "12.00 o'clock, must be time for lunch" habit. It makes no sense to pre-arrange food. Wait till you need it! It's a good idea to skip one meal altogether. If you eat four times a day, drop to three; if you eat three times daily, drop to two. Just forget the usual patterns and so-called regular mealtimes. Maybe your first meal of the day can be at around 11.00 am (by which time your hunger will have built up) Followed by another at around 4.00 pm (which will get you through the evening).

Technically, this comes under the label of *intermittent fasting*, about which more near the end.

4. Don't Eat Unless You Are Really Hungry

This is a variation of #3—don't eat for the sake of routine. It's best to wait till you really need to eat. That feeling of being hungry tells you that you are doing OK on your diet. Put the other way round, if you never feel really hungry, you are overeating!

I don't want you to get into a state where your blood sugar dives and you feel faint, although that may happen at first, while your body adjusts to any diet. The trick is to feel the sensation of hunger is a good thing and a reward, whereas most people dread being hungry and eat before the feeling even comes on.

Relish the feeling of hunger. Yum! It means the plan is working!

5. Shop Differently

You need to cultivate better food buying habits. If you always buy cookies, ice cream, bread and starch foods, you'll eat 'em! You know you will! You need to ban these foods from the house.

Clear the cupboards and pantry of unsuitable foods and stock up with the good stuff. Think about snacks; everyone needs snacks. Just order in a bunch, like grapes, scraped carrots, celery sticks, nuts, etc.

6. Eat Something Good Before You Crave To Eat Something Bad

Fill your cupboards and larder with good, healthy, weight loss foods... and then eat them! Don't wait till you are faint with hunger; you'll probably want to kill for a candy bar. Instead, eat every couple of hours, maximum; just nibble something that's healthy but which will kill your appetite for a while. An apple or a few almonds can give you all the necessary calories for a few hours. You'll need to experiment; we are all different. For example, I find that a nice cup of coffee kills my appetite for anything up to two hours.

7. Home-Cook Your Food...

This one will make you slim AND save you money. Time and again you will notice me say, "Don't eat processed food". This is because so many food industry creations – even 'diet' ones - contain stacks of hidden calories, sugar, salt, trans fats and other really awful stuff. Cook your own meals and you will know what goes into it, plus you are likely to relish the food more if you take time over preparing it.

There's a basic conflict between your needs (eat less) and a restaurant (which wants to sell as much food to you as possible). You'll be under pressure from the start. It's far easier to control your diet by eating at home, even if you have a busy work routine that makes it difficult to do so.

8. Tighten Your Belt

It's an expression we have, for getting used to eating less. It works, though! Wear tighter pants and dresses – resist the temptation to feel comfortable. Feel pinched round the belly, to remind yourself you are on a mission!

9. Motivate Yourself With A Good Photograph Of Your Slimmer Self

Get an old photograph of yourself, back in the days when you were slim and healthy. Put it up on the mirror or refrigerator door, to remind you and inspire you, what you were like when you looked good! Go for it!

10. Eat More! Enjoy More Veggies

The great news is that you never, ever have to go hungry, no matter which weight loss program you are following. You can eat delicious platefuls of fresh vegetables and salads, plus tuck into sublime fruits, knowing that you will still lose weight. Could Nature make it any easier for us? High fiber, high-water content, fewer calories and loads of vital nutrients – it's a total win-win. Just make sure you eat them as close to their natural state as possible, seasoning only with fresh lemon, lime and herbs, not slushy sauces, to gain maximum benefits.

11. Be a Souper-Slimmer

Warm, nourishing and very filling, homemade soup can also be high in nutrients and low in carbs and calories. Forget canned, additive-laden imitations; ignore creamy versions, or those with potatoes in; – go for bright, fresh flavors – chicken and vegetable broth, or exotic Thai soups with shrimp, chili, lemongrass and bok choi are so simple and healthy. Make a large pot of it on Sunday and it will last all week.

12. Aim for those 'Skinny Jeans'

Motivation is vital when losing weight. Find a fabulous piece of clothing that you are longing to be able to get into and use it as your inspiration. It might be a new cocktail dress in a smaller size, or your favorite jeans from 5 years ago. Hang it up, take it out, look at it, and keep trying it on. If you love it enough, keep on track and you'll soon be wearing it!

13. Avoid Sugar At All Costs

Don't be fooled into buying so-called low-fat processed products and drinks which are full of sugar – they will hamper your best efforts. Instead, eat a little fruit when you fancy something sweet and keep your taste buds happy with fresh, interesting spices like cinnamon. Never eat the refined white stuff again. You will not succeed in your diet if you overdose on this highly addictive, calorie-packed substance – see section 8 to find out why sugar is so lethal.

14. Don't Gobble Your Food

When you eat, take your time – what's the hurry? This really is one of the best slimming tips around. Savor each mouthful and make the meal last. If you wish, set a time for 20 minutes and learn how to spread out your enjoyment for longer. It takes 20 minutes for the body to feel full, so wolfing it down in seconds will only fool you into eating more. Slow down to slim.

15. Watch the Drink

Alcohol can trip up many people when they try to follow a diet. A gram of alcohol has 7 calories, while a gram of carbohydrates or protein each has only 4 calories; fat has 9 calories, not much more than alcohol! So be sure to at least cut back, but do be realistic. A complete ban may involve fewer calories but may have you reaching for carb-loaded snacks instead. A glass or two of red wine may even be beneficial, relaxing you (parasympathetic status) and topping up your healthy resveratrol levels.

But watch out for the fact that alcohol can sometimes lower your blood sugar suddenly, which will cause you to feel hungry. That's what cocktails and especially aperitifs are all about: stimulating the appetite!

16. Enjoy Some Herbal Tea

Try a herbal infusion instead! Herb teas can be enjoyed without milk or sugar and green tea can have great health benefits. It has been shown to boost your metabolism, thanks to the phytochemicals called catechins. Plus a nice, hydrating, warming mug of camomile, tulsi or green tea has virtually zero calories and may suppress the appetite. Enjoy it freely.

17. Small Plate, Tall Thin Glass

Cut calories with ease by using the right crockery and glassware. A thin glass will cut your juice or wine intake by up to 30% and a smaller plate will look full and inviting, tempting your eye and helping you to be satisfied with smaller portions! Just this tip alone can help you take off as much as 20 pounds a year.

18. Celebrate Each Victory

Reward yourself as the pounds drop off, to keep yourself motivated—but not with a few pints of beer and a 12-inch pizza, of course! Celebrate in a way that does not sabotage what you are doing – with a beauty treat like a massage or facial, a new pair of shoes (which you can enjoy even as you shed further pounds), or some jewelry. Tell people about your success and be proud of yourself!

19. Don't Eat Your Main Meal Late Into The Evening

Otherwise you just sit around with a ton of unused calories in your stomach before you go to bed. Try to do as the French do and eat a substantial meal for lunch and then very little after that.

Maybe that's the big secret of why French woman are so proverbially slim!

20. Turn Off The TV!

Last but not least, did you now that dining while viewing can make you take in 40 percent more calories than usual? It's proven by research! And texting, driving, or any other distracting activity during a meal can also result in your eating too much. Get rid of distractions and treat eating as a task, not a "treat". It's safer.

But I promised you 21 valuable tips. Let me make sure you understand this last hack is probably the biggest of all:

21. Change Your Tribe!

This is so crucial, you have to understand: IF YOU HANG OUT WITH PEOPLE WHO OVER-EAT HABITUALLY, YOU WILL OVER-EAT TOO. It's inevitable. It's just human nature! So don't do it. If you don't want to change your circle of friends and don't mind seeing yourself really slim and making others around you feel uncomfortable, at least quit eating with them!

Eat alone or—far more effective, as we shall see—cook your own foods, from the advice and fast lessons you'll learn here in this book.

PART 2. THE ISSUES

EVERYTHING THAT CAN INFLUENCE WEIGHT, UP OR DOWN

PART 2. THE ISSUES

SECTION 3.
THE FOOD INDUSTRY IS NOT ON YOUR SIDE!

Before we go any further, let me tell you something important and fundamental: You're on your own. The food industry does not give a damn about your health and your weight, no matter WHAT the label says!

They are out to make a profit and the only way to do this is to hype their unhealthy, dangerous and fattening junk, which they do with tricks and lies. Their artful spin is intended to put over the idea that their products are just as good (or better) than real food.

Most of it has little or no nutritional worth and a lot of it has a negative health impact.

So when you see something labeled as a "diet" product, it is not because it will help you lose weight. *It's because they have found it increases sales (and sometimes even profits) to make such claims.* They rely on trusting customers... oops, almost wrote suckers there... to buy into the lies and suppose the product does what it says, with no downside.

This is helped by a certain gullibility, naivety or—dare I say it, stupidity—on the part of many people, who really want to believe that they are helping their health, or "doing the right thing", whilst continuing to guzzle and slurp modified versions of their favorite food fixes.

I hope you are not one of these cases. But sadly, the number of people who want to remain ignorant and refuse to look at inconvenient truths are by far the majority. It's like the infant's game, "I can't see you, therefore you can't see me," meaning, "If I don't look at the fact that this disgusting, un-healthy, non-nutritious fake food is harming me, then it's perfectly OK to eat it!"

Get Real

As you will read over and over in this book, the only way to permanent weight loss and vibrant health is by adopting the right lifestyle criteria. Just using a "diet" to lose weight and then going back to what you are doing is a foolishness that is doomed to failure.

To be a weight loss hero or heroine, you need to give up all the plasticized, colored, flavor-added, sugary sweet, "enhanced" foods and go back to eating what Nature intended us to eat: wholefoods (meaning real foods, just the way they come).

The only truly safe way to step your way through the minefield of claims, lies, tempting colors and flavors, deliberately addictive synthetic foods and false advertizing, is to give up manufactured food, completely. Just don't eat anything from a packet, jar, tin or bottle and you'll do fine. If it has a list of ingredients, don't eat it!

Apart from the fact that processed foods have been stripped of many vital nutrients during their processing and then had all kinds of inferior, synthetic, bizarre and sometimes just plain toxic ingredients added to them to make up for this shortfall in true flavor and nutritional merit should give every consumer enough reason to stop and think.

Then when you realize that the food peddlers are not content with just trying to sell you their unhealthy wares, they are also eager to get you hooked on them... seriously, *run, don't walk,* in the other direction!

Now's your chance. Just so you can gain some idea of the ludicrous and twisted nature of manufactured foods, consider the next few sections. Read them as if your life depended on the truth; because it does.

The 10 Worst Lies Told About Food Additives and Ingredients

Most of us are trained, at our mother's knee, to believe that food is, by nature, something nourishing, life-giving and necessary. No surprise, because what we ate for thousands of years, straight from the tree or fresh after the hunt, really was nourishing. If it looked fresh and smelled right, we could trust it.

It is only in extremely recent times—the blink of an eye in the context of the million-year timespan of Humankind—that we have started to process and meddle, add and take away from our food, sometimes right up to the point that it becomes completely nutritionally bankrupt.

But we have been slower to unlearn that trust. We have allowed ourselves to be suckered. Our innate friendship with food has been abused. Bad-tasting creations have been masked with additives and extracts not known to Nature, slop that our ancestors would have poured away has been colored pink and sold to us a treat; and we have paid heavily for the privilege of deluding ourselves.

As if that were not outrageous enough, the food industry takes pains to tell us that it really does care. The "diet food" industry is, ironically, one of the worst offenders, trying to claim that their highly processed products could offer any genuinely healthy benefits. Don't believe me? Let's take a look at some of the biggest lies that we, the consumers, are expected to swallow down every day...

1. "Vitamin enriched"

One of the overarching lies and a whopper at that. Big Food companies are claiming to pump vitamins into everything from chocolate chip waffles to margarine and then trying to sell it on as a healthy option. *But what they put in is only a fraction of what they take out!* That's not enrichment; that's robbery!

Think of it this way: if a guy came up to you in the street and robbed you of $100, then gave you back a $5 bill before walking away, would you consider yourself "enriched"? In pretending that the miniscule quantities of artificially added vitamins will turn vitiated (weakened) food into something nourishing, they are trying to pander to the public's wishful-thinking: that you can have your slurpy, sugary junk food and drink and it will still be in some way nourishing. Don't swallow the lie!

Yes, we can live exclusively on sodas and McDonald's burgers. But as Morgan Spurlock showed in his movie *Supersize Me*, in less than thirty days, he was exhausted, his liver was seriously damaged and he started to pile on the pounds. Despite this, McDonald's issued a press release that stated: "There is no question that McDonald's food can fit into a balanced diet, and well within the recommended daily calorie intakes for men and women."

2. "Only 100 calories" (or whatever)

This sort of phrase sounds so tempting, doesn't it? Don't be fooled. You can bet your bottom dollar that these will be 100 empty, highly-refined sugar calories that will send your blood glucose levels soaring, then crash you back down into hunger, whilst giving you nothing beneficial at all. Then you'll crave more (which is what the food producers want). Far better to eat twice as many calories of something that once grew, flew, ran or swam!

3. "Fat-free" or "low-fat"

How can they lie about that, you may wonder? But while on the surface it may be true, it is in fact a massive distraction tactic.

Let's do the math. Suppose a food is claimed to be 99% fat free on the label. It means fat-free *by weight*. But suppose the hypothetical food contains 50 calories and 3 grams of fat. If that is the case, then guess what? Because there are 9 calories per gram of fat, then that means that your low fat food contains 27 calories out of 50. So if you look at the percentage of fat by calories, your low-fat food ends up being over 50% fat!

Also, get this: since fat gives food a lot of flavor, manufacturers have to do something to make the food taste better when they remove it. So they add salt, high fructose corn syrup, modified food starch (GMO origins), free glutamates (MSG, hydrolyzed vegetable protein and natural flavors), diglycerides (sugar) and gums (guar and xanthan). These often add more calories and carbs than the fat calories you are supposedly avoiding!

4. "With added iron"

I know you will find it hard to believe that manufacturers would ever add actual iron filings to cereal just so they could boast that it contained 100% of your iron RDA. But they do... Iron filings are not bioavailable and in fact may represent a toxic form of iron ("hot" iron, a damaging oxidative species)... so you had better watch this video by Thomas E. Levy MD: http://youtu.be/OMNxya1QZQI

5. "Organic" (for highly processed food)

Organic is good, of course. But what makes me mad is seeing the organic label slapped onto products that will clog up your system with highly processed trash that you could do without. Like the packets of 'organic' macaroni cheese you can buy with high-sodium, high-sugar, high-fat powdered cheese and a mountain of starchy carbs. It may not contain pesticides, but it is not at all organic (which means nature-made) and is sure going to play havoc with your body. Junk is junk, even if free of pesticides.

6. "No cholesterol"

Another cunning distraction tactic. It commonly appears on labels of foods which have no dairy content, but plenty of other baddies like lots of sugar. Trying to avoid dietary cholesterol is a fool's game. Your body makes more cholesterol internally than you could possibly swallow.

Anyway, as I have written elsewhere, the body needs a certain amount of cholesterol to be healthy. The fraudulent work of Ancel Keys, targeting fats, has been exposed at last and there is no longer any reason to fear saturated fat. It's *oxidized* fat that harms your arteries. Hence the need to take plentiful anti-oxidants (colored foods).

7. "Made with real...(whatever)"

This one is very clever. We want to feed our kids suppers that have nuggets that are 'made with real chicken' right? Wrong! It will technically be true that a percentage of the product will have been made with actual poultry but all too often, when you investigate further, the 'real' food sits alongside flavorings, additives, processed soy protein, modified food starch and much more.

The words "made with" are a trick, to get you to believe it's entirely 100% real chicken, whereas as it is really only "made with some... included." A moment's reflection will enable you to see that if it's manufactured, it is altered. Otherwise just buy a real chicken and cook it yourself!

8. "Diet soda

It may be low on calories (because it's low of food value) but it certainly isn't good for your diet, as the name tries to suggest. It provides insufficient nutritional benefits, bar the hydration from its contained water that you would be better off drinking in its purest form. Plus, the phosphoric acid that can be found in many colas may leach calcium from your bones, ultimately leading to osteoporosis. We are seeing young girls these days, some even in their 20s, who have a degree of osteoporosis equivalent to a seventy year old, due to drinking excessive soda drinks.

9. "Low sugar"

We all know too much sugar is bad for us, what harm could this product do? That depends on which artificial chemical the product has been crammed full of instead. Aspartame and sucralose (Splenda) are substances that should never enter the human body. Safety claims are all faked. There simply has not been sufficient safety testing. The FDA supposedly reviewed 110 studies, before approving sucralose BUT, out of these 110 studies, only two were human studies, and *the longest one was conducted for four days*! [1]

10. "Zero grams trans fats"

Let's end with a biggie. It's one of the few times that the food industry gives you something for 'nothing' and, unfortunately, it's a potential killer of a lie. The FDA lets manufacturers claim that their products contain 'Zero gram trans fats' when in fact they mean they contain less than 0.5 gram of trans fats per serving. Firstly, they pick what 'a serving' is and in some cases make it as little as a spoonful! Then, legally, every eating portion could have as much as 5 grams (0.49 for compliance) of trans fat. That could be a horrendous amount of trans fats you are eating, while being told there is none in the food!

That's right; zero does not mean zero at all! Thanks to this trickery, the amount of cheap, dangerous, synthetic fats you consume can rapidly add up and the industry knows that, so they try to hide the fact entirely that they are in your food.

One of the food industry's greatest cons is to conjure up the idea that their highly processed snacks are 'just like Momma used to make'. So they tell us that their popcorn, say, is made with a 'taste of butter'. Can't you just see that butter churn on the home ranch... Look again! This 'butter' is in fact partially hydrogenated yellow-dyed soybean oil comprising many grams of deadly trans fats. *Some popular brands of popcorn contain over 7 times what you should safely consume in a day, by the standards of the American Heart Association.*

Starting to see a picture? It's all lies, half-truths, tricks and distraction tactics! But we know better. Right?

They Get You Addicted To Carbs

You may often hear people who struggle with their weight try to explain their predicament:

"I can't resist, I'm just addicted to chocolate cake/chips/white bread..."

We nod and sympathize, but hold on... when was the last time someone said to you "I'm addicted to spinach" or "I have a serious tuna problem?"

We would laugh out loud because we know that, whilst we may really love fish, vegetables or other healthy foods and ideally eat a lot of them, it is almost exclusively a positive relationship we have with that food. Why, then, do we instinctively feel that we might respond differently to starchy carbohydrates, those foods with a high glycemic index?

The answer is that we genuinely do—they truly are addictive!

A recent study found that highly-processed carbohydrates (high glycemic index) can affect pleasure and addiction centers in the brain. In other words, there are strong similarities in the way respond to a bag of potato chips and, for example, cocaine.

The study had two overweight groups of men consume milkshakes that were almost identical except that one type had a high-glycemic index (GI) and one was low-glycemic.

High-glycemic carbohydrates—white bread, pasta, rice, cakes—are quickly digested, whereas low-glycemic carbs—most fruits, vegetables, whole grains—take much longer to digest.

Four hours after they had consumed the milkshakes, the subjects of the experiment were given fMRI brain scans that measured brain activity.

Those subjects who had drunk the high GI shakes had a surge in blood sugar, which then crashed predictably four hours later (see section 8). By the time the scan took place, not only did they experience a raging hunger, but the fMRIs showed "intense" activity in the *nucleus accumbens*, a region of the brain which is involved in addiction.

Those who drank the low GI shakes did not experience the same hunger or show this brain activity, even though the shakes had a similar number of calories and sweetness. It was the GI factor that made the difference and high GI carbs were shown to be addictive, which could lead to over-eating. [2]

This study makes explicit what I have always believed: that high glycemic index foods do not satisfy our appetites but actually cause hunger and we eat more!

There is, inarguably, a direct link between the fact that the US is suffering from an obesity epidemic and at the same time the USDA issues guidelines that not only insists that carbs are healthy but says that they should make up the majority of the food we eat; up to 65 percent of all calories! It doesn't make any sense!

We can get more than enough carbohydrate from green vegetables, fruit and other healthy foodstuffs. Nature really has got it covered so we can ditch the crazy advice, which is there to support the farmers, not you!

MSG Is Highly Addictive (As Well As Toxic)

For some years we have been aware that mono-sodium glutamate, or MSG, is pretty toxic stuff—literally. Present in an enormous number of processed foods and used to enhance flavor, it has in fact been proven to be an 'excitotoxin' or neurotoxin that has a degenerative effect on the brain and nervous system, even though the FDA call it a GRAS ('generally recognized as safe'). The fact that it is a toxin certainly doesn't make it sound delicious does it?

The truth is that food manufacturers know that many of us have fallen into the MSG addiction trap and will therefore keep coming back for more, over and over.

But you may be surprised to learn that MSG has also been pinpointed as a major cause of obesity.

Like many other excitotoxins, monosodium glutamate causes a response in the body that runs something like: insulin spike, then an adrenalin rush, fat storage and then craving more food. This endlessly unsatisfying vicious circle is the origin of the most famous takeaway food puzzle:

'Why is it that when you eat Chinese food, you feel hungry an hour later?'

It is no coincidence that Chinese food is a cuisine that widely uses the addition of MSG 'enhance' the flavor. More and more people have noticed over the years that Chinese food leaves you relatively unsatisfied, despite the delicious flavor.

If you stick to unprocessed, home-cooked food you should have no problem avoiding MSG, but on the occasions when you do by a food product that has a label, read it carefully. MSG peddlers like to play hide and seek!

One of the tricks they use is to disguise its presence by changing the name. Knowing that just about everyone hates MSG and is wary of it, manufacturers use other labels instead like hydrolyzed vegetable protein (HVP), textured protein, monopotassium glutamate, hydrolyzed plant protein (HPP), autolyzed plant protein, yeast extract, autolyzed yeast and vegetable protein extract, vetsin, ajinomoto and umami.

You need to learn to spot these phoney cover-up names. Avoid them all, they're just MSG! But there's more...

One study fed rats large amounts of MSG over an extended period of time. The report declared that the amount of adrenaline, dopamine and serotonin that the rats produced went up significantly as their adrenal gland grew in weight. By 60 weeks of age the MSG-fed rats had developed a form of Type II diabetes.[3]

There it is again, another way of ultimately flooding the brain with the same chemicals as if we were taking a hit of Class A drugs! It's a double whammy; a food that triggers pleasure in the brain and the food industry's Holy Grail, because it actually makes you hungry.

Yes, a food ingredient that makes you think it tastes good but is actually a toxin; food that does the opposite of what food should—it actually makes you hungry and keeps you coming back for more. Is it any wonder that we are in the middle of an obesity epidemic?

The Final Shattering Secret of Monosodium Glutamate

I'm not finished yet. There is one more layer of trouble with MSG in foods... It's a shocking and closely guarded secret.

We've seen that people who eat more MSG are more likely to be overweight or obese. BUT IT'S NOT JUST BECAUSE THEY ARE EATING MORE. The shocking fact has emerged that, eating the same foods, calorie for calorie, individuals allowing MSG into their bodies will increase in weight, over individuals who do not eat the MSG.

In other words, *add in the MSG and you gain weight, even on the same number of calories.* That's startling, even for me.

Scientists (and their promoters) want it downplayed and "it's not a big difference" they say. Well, that's phoney, because MSG foods are just about universal and, unless you are careful to avoid it, you eat MSG every single meal, in some form or other. There is a cumulative effect.

In the latest research, published in the *American Journal of Clinical Nutrition*, men and women who ate the most MSG (around 5 grams a day) were about 30 percent more likely to become overweight by the end of the study than those who ate the least amount of the flavoring (less than a half-gram a day). In fact, after excluding people who were overweight at the start of the study, the risk rose to 33 percent.

Why MSG and weight gain may be linked isn't clear but is most probably due to the discovery that people who consumed more MSG produced more leptin. MSG consumption may thus lead to leptin resistance and over eating (see section 9). [4]

Ghastly Yuck. "I'd Never Eat That!" But Actually You Do...

Still believe that processed food products are mostly pretty wholesome and, as they often like to claim, 'full of natural goodness' (another made-up phrase with rarely any basis in truth when food has been processed)?

Well, they're certainly full of something, but perhaps not what you believe. None of us would really choose to eat some of the truly disgusting ingredients that have been cunningly packed inside a strawberry-flavored pudding or hot dog. But thanks to handing control over what we eat to an industry that does not care for our health, we do eat a lot of unbelievably disgusting so-called ingredients, every time we buy a processed product.

A few of the worst offenders are:

1. Beaver's Butt

I doubt you have ever licked a beaver's ass. But then again, maybe you've often come close, without realizing it! Anal gland secretions from beavers, called *Castoreum*, smells like vanilla and are used to flavor baked goods, pudding, chewing gum and more. Have you ever imagined that you would be happy to put the secretions from around a beaver's anus into your mouth? And who dreamed up the name *Castoreum*, to hide its origins?

All we know is that few people would consider it food and most people would agree that eating it is a pretty gross thought. Worst of all, it may not even show up as *Castoreum* on the ingredients list, just as 'natural flavoring'. Talk about poetic license!

2. Wood Pulp

Tiny pieces of plant fibers and wood called powdered cellulose are used to make some types of low-fat ice cream seem more creamy. It's also used to prevent some shredded cheese from clumping.

3. Ammonia

Yes, actual ammonia; the chemical with the overpowering violent odor that is commonly found in household cleaning products. Unfortunately, the geniuses in the food industry also think it is great to use it as a gas to kill the germs in their cheap, filthy, bacteria-laden trimmed meat. This turns it into 'pink slime' (don't worry, we're coming to that)...

Ammonia is not food. Don't take anyone's word for it, just remember that caveman sense of smell we all used to rely on. Does the smell of ammonia say to you 'eat this, it's good?' Of course not!

4. Crushed Insects (carmine or cochineal beetle)

Mouth-watering, right? The crushed, boiled cochineal beetles are very widely used in the food industry to supply a bright red food-coloring. They use it in ice cream, sweets, drinks and more. Many people are seriously allergic to the bugs and even sustain anaphylactic reactions to this false food.

5. Antifreeze (ethylene glycol)

More food industry madness. Ethylene glycol has been used as a poison to murder someone in more than one case. Think of what antifreeze does to your iced up windscreen and imagine an active ingredient of that in your stomach. Not nice.

6. Shellac (furniture polish!)

Want to know what the lovely shiny coating is on the outside of some sugar-laden favorites such as certain jelly beans? There is an insect that lives in Thailand called the *Kerria lacca*, the female of which makes sticky secretions called shellac. That is what you're eating. The ever-inventive food industry often calls it 'confectioner's glaze' as if it were handmade by a twinkly-eyed candy-creator. Note: it is exactly the same stuff that's dissolved in alcohol to make French furniture polish!

7. Antibiotics

We get more antibiotics second-hand in our food than as medicines. This class of miracle drugs has slowly been rendered worthless by the creation of resistance strains of bacteria, 80% of which is due to commercial abuse. Antibiotics are used to make livestock into fatter commodities faster, then we eat the meat pumped full of drugs we didn't ask for. Antibiotic-resistant bacteria proliferate, more people get sick from delights such as resistant salmonella and we are left with yet another dangerous mess in the food chain.

8. Phosphates

Phosphates are naturally present in food. We now know they are a health hazard, particularly for someone with inadequate kidney function. Substances called polyphosphates are injected into chicken, ham and other foodstuffs. These chemicals bind with water and add bulk. The legal limit for faking food "weight" in this way is around 40% by weight (depends on the country).

You will notice this effect when cooking bacon or ham; once heated, liquid starts to emerge from the slices, which then shrivel to maybe half the volume. You are sold water, just to plump up food and make more money, you understand. Goodbye natural food, hello high blood pressure.

Food products with high phosphate contents are damaging to the health of the general public, and as such should be labeled, say researchers behind a new study. [5]

9. Viruses

Yes, viruses are sometimes deliberately added to foods. Bacteriophages, tiny viruses that attack and kill bacteria, are used in instances where food such as deli meats, are sold in plastic pouches, they are designed to combat E. coli. Approved as recently as 2006, who knows the long-term impact on our bodies that they may prove to have? One thing is for sure: viruses mutate unpredictably. What may be safe at one time could turn into a deadly pathogen.

Why add bacteriophages to food? To combat filthy practices within the food industry.

10. Finally "Pink Slime"

If you are still a step away from feeling totally nauseated by food industry practices, hold on! We must not forget the ingredient with its rightful horror-comic name 'Pink Slime'. It is even worse than its name. Pink slime is created when bits of meat which are still clinging to fat are recovered by melting away the fat and spinning the results in a centrifuge. The pink slime, as if not ugly enough already, is then treated with ammonia gas (see item 3) to kills germs. Tasty.

Still can't picture how bad this stuff really is? It is so very disgusting that I had to give you a couple of images to see how your most basic hunter-gather sense of sight reacts to two spot-the-difference images.

This is what is organic, grass-fed beef, the very best source of Omega-3s, an outstanding source of Acetyl L-Carnitine (ALC) and rich in protein looks like: http://bit.ly/1eA908T

This is what mechanically separated pink gloop "meat" looks like: http://bit.ly/1ezRKjS

Which one would you pick? (thank you to health.com)

Do Genetically Modified Foods Make Us Fat?

I'm putting GMO foods into this section, even though, strictly speaking, they are an abomination of the agricultural industry, rather than food manufacturers.

Nevertheless, Big Food knows what it is doing with the product. They are in cahoots with Big Ag and use their products indiscriminately, for one reason only: more profit.

GMO foods don't just make you fat; they will inflame your tissues, shorten your life and definitely cause cancer.

First, the weight gain issue. A study published in the *International Journal of Biological Sciences* shows that eating GMO food is almost certainly contributing to the obesity epidemic. GMO foods cause inflammation and in this important book, I spare no opportunity to repeatedly remind you that inflammation leads to obesity problems (section 7). [6]

But I'm not just limiting my warnings to the weight gain issue. The test animals also showed increases in circulating glucose and triglycerides plus significant damage to major organs. Effects were mostly associated with the kidney and liver, the dietary detoxifying organs, but other effects were also noticed in the heart, adrenal glands, spleen and hematopoietic (blood making) system.

So overall health suffers too.

GMO foods are significant contributors to the diabetes and obesity epidemic.

Now learn this: in another shocking study, pigs fed a diet of genetically engineered soy and corn showed a 267% increase in severe stomach inflammation compared to those fed non-GMO diets. In males, the difference was even more pronounced: a 400% increase. So the fact that GMO foods are inflammatory in nature is now beyond question.

The study was carried out over a 23-week period by eight researchers across Australia and the USA and was published in the *Journal of Organic Systems*, a peer-reviewed science journal.[7]

Of course the study was quickly attacked by the food industry; that's quite standard. They put their paid shill scientists on it, to try and find details to criticize. For them there must never be any acknowledgement of possible dangers from GMO foods... never, never, never.

To keep up their standpoint, all they have to do is ignore the gathering tide of evidence or lie about it. They do both very well.

The usual bluster and denial tactics were used against another powerful and disturbing report published in 2012, also in a peer-reviewed journal: *Food and Chemical Toxicology*. The world was shocked by hideous photographs of rats fed on grains engineered to be tolerant of Monsanto's infamous "Roundup" pesticide, bearing grotesque tumors that had grown in just a matter of a few months.[8]

The implications for humans are appalling. With GMO foods deliberately hidden in our supply chain, we face the likelihood of eating them for many years to come, maybe generations to come, and growing similar cancers. The trouble is, it will take a long time for the truth to emerge and by then millions of individuals will have been doomed to a miserable death, just for corporate profits.

But yet again, the study was cynically and systematically attacked. Seralini's own website counters every single twisted and dishonest objection.

Here are 10 points on which industry criticisms are false:

1. That Séralini's study was a badly designed cancer study. It wasn't. It was a chronic toxicity study – and a well-designed and well-conducted one. The cancers were what happened to show up.

2. Séralini's study is the only long-term study on the commercialized GMO maize NK603 and the pesticide (Roundup) it is designed to be grown with.

3. Séralini used the same strain of rat (Sprague-Dawley, SD) that Monsanto used in its 90-day studies on GMO foods and its long-term studies on glyphosate, the chemical ingredient of Roundup, conducted for regulatory approval.

4. Despite wild claims to the contrary, the SD rat is about as prone to tumors as humans are. As with humans, the SD rat's tendency to cancer increases with age.

5. Compared with industry tests on GMO foods, Séralini's study analyzed the same number of rats but over a longer period (two years instead of 90 days), measured more effects more often, and was uniquely able to distinguish the effects of the GMO food from the pesticide it is grown with.

6. If we argue that Séralini's study does not prove that the GMO food tested is dangerous, then we must also accept that industry studies on GM foods cannot prove they are safe.

7. Séralini's study showed that 90-day tests commonly done on GMO foods are not long enough to see long-term effects like cancer, organ damage, and premature death. The first tumors only appeared 4-7 months into the study.

8. Séralini's study showed that industry and regulators are wrong to dismiss toxic effects seen in 90-day studies on GMO foods as "not biologically meaningful". Signs of toxicity found in Monsanto's 90-day studies were found to develop later into organ damage, cancer, and premature death in Séralini's two-year study.

9. Long-term tests on GMO foods are not required by regulators anywhere in the world.

10. GMO foods have been found to have toxic effects on laboratory and farm animals in a number of other studies. This is not a "one-off" finding.[9]

The sad fact remains that the journal *Food and Chemical Toxicology* was eventually forced by Monsanto and other vested interests to withdraw its publication of Seralini's work. The specious argument used was that it followed a "flawed" cancer study protocol. But it wasn't a cancer study at all! It was a toxicology study, conducted by one of the world's leading scientists, using impeccable toxicology research protocols.

But now the food industry can breathe easily once again: apparently there were no tumors growing on the test animals after all!

Government Collusion

The truth is we and our governments are being tricked and manipulated by a wall of lies to cover up quite serious crimes against humanity. It's the biotech industry versus the human race.

Keep your eye on the alternative press and activist websites like InfoWars.com and NaturalNews.com—they fight hard to make public the hidden lies, corruption and deceitful agenda of the biotech industry. Otherwise you risk being left in the dark.

[*at the time of writing, these two websites have been blocked by Google, meaning the crooks that own and run Google don't want you to see the facts you are entitled to*]

The USA is the largest producer of genetically modified crops. But more than a dozen other countries around the world have latched on to the technology, including Argentina, Canada, China, Australia, India, and Mexico.

You could be eating GM foods and not even know it. A USDA-funded survey, reported by WebMD, shows you're not alone. Researchers from the Food Policy Institute at Rutgers' Cook College found that only 52% of Americans realized that genetically modified foods have already entered the supply chain and are being sold in grocery stores. Everyone else is ignorant of the fact.

Europe, of course, has continued to fight against GMO foods. But these hazards are entering our food chain by stealth. There is nothing to stop a bird from ingesting GMO seeds in one country and then pooping on someone else's land, where individuals may feel "safe" from GMO invasion.

Yet the FDA effects not to be concerned and holds to the line that these foods are totally safe. The recommendation that GMO food be labeled for what it is, so people could make an informed choice, is rejected: "Genetically modified" is an inappropriate term, in that all crop varieties have been modified by plant breeders, is the absurd FDA claim.

According to a WebMD feature article, the most common genetically modified foods are soybeans, maize (corn), cotton, and rapeseed oil. That means many foods made in the U.S. containing corn or high-fructose corn syrup, such as many breakfast cereals, snack foods, and the last soda you drank; foods made with soybeans (including some baby foods); and foods made with cottonseed and canola oils could likely have genetically modified ingredients.[10]

Then there are secondary foods. Chocolate, for instance, could contain at least a few GMO ingredients: high fructose corn syrup from GMO corn, sugar from GMO beets, and soy lecithin from GMO soy. Soy lecithin is an emulsifier that keeps the chocolate solid and gives it a longer shelf life.

Meat is indirectly contaminated. Chicken, pigs, and cows that eat unnatural GMO feed become GMO themselves. To make matters worse, a study out of Italy shows that the GMO feed that animals eat even affects the milk they produce.

According to the study, genetically-modified DNA from corn was present in 25% of milk samples. Even if you steer clear of GMO foods, your animal products may be passing their synthetic diet along to you.

How To Avoid GM

This text is not about the politics of food and agri-business. But those of us in the know feel very sure that some of our worsening obesity problems (and possibly other rapidly growing issues, like autism) could well be due the consumption of GMO foods.

You need to be alert to avoid them if at all possible.

And I say "if possible", because in the USA, you can't; it's too late. The supply line is already irretrievably contaminated. Even supposed GMO-free crops by now have become contaminated by cross-pollination with DNA from adjacent GMO fields. Short of blowing every bird and bug out of the atmosphere, this cross-contamination process will continue relentlessly.

Try to buy only quality organic, raw, grass fed, or naturally pastured foods. Buy the best you can with "certified organic", which can itself be a scam. But it's important to understand that even when you think you're eating "all natural," that food is probably as far from natural as you can get. And it may be full of GMO ingredients.

Buying organic may cost more. But the higher price tag often comes with a greater peace of mind. Just don't think you are totally safe, is all.

PART 2. THE ISSUES

SECTION 4. HORMONES WHICH REGULATE APPETITE

Say what? The idea of hunger being controlled in any way by hormones might seem a little counter-intuitive at first. But in fact several hormones have emerged which regulate appetite in one direction or another (up or down) and it seems likely that more are waiting to be discovered.

A hormone is a signaling molecule that has an effect in very small amounts indeed (way below any obvious biochemical quantities). The key to their effect is the presence of special receptors in the target tissue, which are acutely sensitive and tuned to their particular hormone, like a short-wave radio tuned to a particular station. If someone is transmitting that waveband anywhere on Earth—atmospheric conditions permitting—a keen amateur radio ham can pick up the signal and understand what is being said, even if the signal intensity is vanishingly small.

So it is with hormones, a tiny presence can produce very large effects.

There are direct and indirect hormones affecting metabolism and weight gain. For example insulin, the glucose control hormone has an direct bearing on fat storage. Also thyroid hormones, which up-regulate metabolism, causing the body engine to run faster or slower on the same calorie intake, will have a profound effect on weight.

I have said elsewhere and repeat in this book that low thyroid function is one of the most disastrously under-diagnosed medical pathologies in the world. I have also explained why (page 134).

But in this section we will concentrate our attention on a small group of hormone substances which seem to directly affect appetite. Several of these are adipokines, meaning they are secreted directly from fat cells, or adipocytes. So if there is less fat tissue, less fat cells, these hormones will diminish in the blood.

Let's start with one of the best known:

Leptin

Leptin is a true adipokine, secreted exclusively by fat cells in the body. It suppresses the appetite, which is useful. When it was discovered, pharmaceutical companies went into overdrive, dreaming of the trillions of dollars that could be made, by marketing a hormone which suppresses a person's appetite!

Unfortunately (for us all, not just for the drug companies), it was quickly found that obese and overweight individuals have excess levels of leptin. They didn't need any more... their body was not listening to the leptin signal, which went up and up and up... and was still being ignored; a condition we call *leptin resistance*.

You would be right to think this sounds a bit like insulin resistance, which most people have heard of and even seem to understand; insulin is a good thing to have around but when there is way too much of it, then it means the body isn't paying attention to it. High insulin levels point to a real failure of blood sugar control and is one of the most definite markers of early death, if not THE number one marker.

Leptin resistance is turning out to be pretty deadly too. When an obese person's metabolism fails to listen to the hormone which cries "Stop eating!" this is likely to lead to spiraling calorie intake, raised blood sugar, increased tissue fat deposits and... yes, early death again.

But it's worse than just the weight gain. It's been found that leptin is actually what we call an inflammatory cytokine, meaning its mere presence raises inflammation levels in the body. Inflammation is the number one ager and killer, so that's a very deadly side-effect.

We need to get leptin levels DOWN and to have our bodies start listening to that all-important appetite suppression effect. There is only one known way to do that: lose weight!

The more weight you lose, the less leptin. Remember, leptin is secreted by fat cells. So when levels drop to the normal range, your body starts listening to it and obeying the message, which is: stop eating.

Ghrelin

Next let's look at the opposite number, as it were, a hormone which increases the feeling of hunger; an appetite stimulant in other words. Ghrelin promotes positive energy balance by decreasing glucose and fat oxidation and increasing energy storage. The funny name is derived from **gr**owth **h**ormone

release **in**ducing but that's too technical to bother us here. It was first identified in 1999 by Japanese researchers.

Unlike adipokines, ghrelin is secreted by the gut (stomach, small and large intestines), not fat cells (adipocytes).

Ghrelin levels increase before meals and decrease after meals, which is what you would expect for a substance which stimulates the appetite. In certain bariatric procedures (gastric bypass), the level of ghrelin is reduced in patients, thus causing satiation before it would normally occur, which is helpful.[1]

Injections of ghrelin in both humans and rats have been shown to increase food intake in a dose dependent manner. So the more ghrelin that is injected the more food that is consumed. However, ghrelin does not increase meal size, only the frequency of eating. [2]

Humans injected with ghrelin and then allowed open access to food, buffet-style, ate 30% more calories.

However, surprisingly, ghrelin levels are often low in obese individuals; you might expect the opposite to be the case. It is also high in anorexia disturbed individuals—but they have obviously learned to switch off or ignore its signal.

Fortunately, ghrelin has definite anti-inflammatory properties so, in that respect too, it is the opposite of leptin.

But we are not done yet...

Adiponectin

Adiponectin is also a hunger hormone, which interacts with leptin in controlling appetite and has several beneficial properties for us, including enhancing muscle's ability to use carbohydrates for energy, boosting metabolism, increasing the rate of fat breakdown and curbing appetite.

I have already mentioned the role of so-called adipokines, a fancy word just meaning inflammatory substances secreted by fat cells (adipocytes). There is no longer any doubt that these inflammatory substances create a destructive cascade effect, leading to relentless damage of our blood vessels and leading inexorably to heart disease, stroke and death.

Fortunately, adiponectin is also very protective against inflammation. Adiponectin is secreted by the fat cells, or adipocytes, and is important in energy metabolism and insulin resistance. Many obese people have low adiponectin levels and this is associated with the increased risk of developing type 2 diabetes, regardless of body mass index.

Adiponectin levels go down with obesity and surge back as you lose weight. That's another very good reason to want to dump adipose tissue (fat) and live longer.

It has been indicated, in certain animal models, that adiponectin can play a key role in reversing insulin resistance: when combined with leptin in studies it has completely reversed insulin resistance in mice. [3]

Adiponectin is, therefore a vital hormonal friend, particularly for those seeking to lose weight. With regard to increasing levels of adiponectin, there is a popular herbal extract called berberine, which has been shown to promote its production. This is an important aspect of the AMPK "fat switch" mechanism (section 6). Also, when mice were fed certain Omega-3 fatty acids (EPA and DHA), their adiponectin levels increased. That could explain why omega-3 fatty acids are so protective against inflammation.

Estrogen

Not often named as a hunger hormone. But consider this:

Sex hormones fluctuate throughout the month, depending on the menstrual cycle and whether the woman takes a hormonal birth control pill. In general, estrogen is at its lowest on day one of the cycle. It climbs for two weeks, then takes a dive in weeks three and four. Falling estrogen causes serotonin levels to drop and cortisol to rise, so a person may feel cranky and hungrier than usual—which can lead to bingeing, especially on fatty, salty, or sugary foods.

Remember, in this world of estrogen dominance (due to xenoestrogen pollutants in our food and water supplies), men too are affected by estrogen and can suffer these same symptoms; just not cyclically. We'll look at estrogen dominance later.

Meanwhile, don't give yourself a hard time because of temptation and weaknesses. Until you understand and can master the workings of this quartet of hormones, you will often be plagued by inappropriate hunger, and not understand why.

As ever, eating the right nutrients can have a direct bearing on every aspect of our health, including the production of weight-loss supporting hormones. Eating clean, nutrient-dense protein, fat, fiber, and greens helps you eat to satiety. Just stay away from carbs, which wreak havoc with hunger hormones. You'll be satisfied, full, not just for an hour, but easily able to last four to six hours without crashing, craving, or even thinking about food.

Can You Catch Obesity?

Just to introduce an element of confusion, and to show you how interesting and complicated biology can get, let me briefly mention viruses that can cause obesity.

In a study done by Wayne State University, scientists discovered that the human (Ad-36) was found to be linked to obesity in test animals by inhibiting leptin production. We have seen already that leptin is the appetite control hormone that switches OFF the desire to eat.

The inevitable result of leptin lack (or leptin resistance) is over-eating, obesity, increased insulin resistance and the whole nine yards of fat storage.

The preliminary study found that 15 percent of obese people have antibodies to the Ad-36, indicating they were exposed to it, but that no people of average weight did.

"This is the first link of a human virus with human obesity," said Nikhil Dhurandhar, a research scientist who conducted the study with Professor Richard Atkinson, an endocrinologist and nationally known obesity expert.[4]

Trouble is, Ad-36 may not be the only micro-organism capable of this or similar effects.

Dr. Nikhil V. Dhurandhar has devoted his research, at the Pennington Biomedical Research Center, to exploring possible links between micro-organisms, especially viruses and weight gain.

Seven viruses have been reported to be the causes of obesity in animal models by various research groups. It is exciting to think there may be a possible future in which we can prevent virus-related obesity.

Just remember that association is not causation. In other words the frequent presence of a virus where there is a health problem does not mean it is sure to be a culprit.

There is one quick way to downgrade virus infections and it is interesting: electrical currents. Controversial electrical wizard Bob Beck had been obese but lost 145 pounds in a few months by (he claimed) getting rid of the obesity virus with the use of his blood electrification unit. Beck had previously tried all different kinds of diets, including being injected with pregnant mares urine. Beck has now passed on but he believed electro-medicine is a viable alternative treatment to cure overweight caused by the adenovirus known as Ad-36. He said that 40% of the overweight people who used his protocol lost all the weight they wanted to lose. [5]

Japanese white Mulberry extract (*Morus indica*) has been shown to reduce Adenovirus 36 replication in mice. It brought about a reduction in weight and in pro-inflammatory cytokines. Mulberry is also very helpful for blocking sugar metabolism, as we will see in section 8). We are waiting for a study that looks at mulberry extract in humans in reference to adenovirus Ad-36. Meantime, you can try it for yourself. You don't need a prescription!

Check out further properties of mulberry in section 13 (brown adipose tissue).

Chromium

OK, before we wrap it up with appetite control, let's look at one other factor.

It's a trace mineral and is important for the control of blood sugar. Without it, diabetics struggle to keep their numbers in a healthy range. I'm talking about trivalent chromium. This is not the shiny stuff you find on a car radiator grill; I'm referring to organically available chromium.

Only small amounts of trivalent chromium are needed, hence the term "trace element", which is often used to describe this class of nutrients (selenium is another good example).

Chromium controls your appetite, and helps manage food cravings, especially for sweets. It may help you lose fat while you build up lean muscle when used as part of diet and exercise program.

This trace mineral also plays an essential role in the metabolism of carbohydrates and fats and has been shown to promote cardiovascular health. It is speculated that chromium increases the body's sensitivity to insulin (always a good thing, since obesity and insulin resistance go hand in hand).

You'll find claims all over the Internet for the supposed weight loss miracles this supplement can provide, with names like "Ripped Action", "Fat Burner Bars" and "Ripped Fast". Just view most of it with caution. As I always say, "Beware the science from someone who is trying to sell you something!"

Does It Really Work?

In a word, "yes and no" (joke). I mean it does something but not that much. It's most distinctive action is to help switch fat to lean muscle. [6]

Dr. Gil Kaats and a team of researchers from the Health and Medical Research Foundation and the University of Texas Health Science Center studied over 150 people to see if they would lose fat just from taking chromium.

After three months, the group taking the placebo showed no changes. The chromium group lost between 3.4 and 4.6 pounds of body fat. The chromium group also gained an average of 1.4 pounds of lean muscle. [7]

These are trivial changes, compared to those attainable by the other methods described in this book. So, I wouldn't suggest you take chromium in any form and expect to lose much weight. Just take it because your body needs it for optimum health and it can help with your appetite.

Where Do I Get It? Chromium is a naturally-occurring mineral, found in trace amounts in everyday foods like meat, poultry, fish, and whole-grain breads. When foods are processed, they are stripped of natural chromium, making Western diets generally very low in chromium. In 1968, animal studies showed that when adequate levels of chromium are lacking, insulin is not optimally effective, and damage to insulin-dependent systems can occur. [8]

It is generally agreed that the piccolinate form (chromium piccolinate) is best absorbed and does the most good. Go for supplements with 200 mcg.

The current FDA recommended daily chromium intake is 130 mcg. For labelling purposes, the European Union's Recommended Daily Allowance (EU RDA) for chromium has been set lower at 40 mcg per day for adults. The European Food Safety Authority states "up to 250 mcg", however many sources suggest that up to 1,000 mcg a day will be safe for most people. Don't get your mcg mixed up with milligrams, which is 1,000 times more concentrated.

Side Effects

Chromium seems to have few side effects. There have been some reports of chromium causing occasional irregular heartbeats, sleep disturbances and allergic reactions. Chromium may increase the risk of kidney or liver damage. If you have kidney or liver disease, do not take chromium without talking to your GP first.

Interactions. Since chromium may affect blood sugar levels, it is crucial that anyone taking diabetes medications, like Metformin or insulin, only use chromium under medical supervision.

Chromium may also interact with medicines like antacids, acid reflux drugs, corticosteroids, beta-blockers, insulin and NSAID painkillers. These interactions may cause the chromium to be poorly absorbed or amplify the effect of the medication being taken. I repeat: work with your doctor on this (but make him or her take action!)

PART 2. THE ISSUES

SECTION 5. FOOD ALLERGIES AND ADDICTION

This section is not about HOW MUCH you eat; it's about WHAT you eat. There's a crucial difference. If you drop out certain foods, regardless of calorie values, you'll lose weight, if it's an allergy food. Similarly, if you eat an allergy food, even with almost no calories (I've seen it with black coffee, for instance), you'll gain weight.

Tracking down these weight-gain allergens will make life very easy for you, because you can eat all you want of the healthy safe foods!

Just one word of warning, however: there are no hard-and-fast food allergens. To read the nonsense by self-styled experts on the web, you'd think all you had to worry about was casein and gluten; avoid those and you're done. This is very silly.

I have seen allergic reactions to just about any food you can name: even lettuce, carrots, tomatoes and almonds. This chapter is an early milestone, to help you settle this aspect of dietary intolerance. For many individuals it was the only discovery they needed to lose weight quickly, eliminate chronic symptoms, and to look and feel ten to fifteen years younger.

You'll learn about the mechanism of hidden food allergies, which my late friend Amelia Nathan-Hill (founder of the charity "Action Against Allergy") christened "the unsuspected enemy".

You'll also learn how to test yourself for hidden food allergies. This is far more accurate than the usual blood tests or dowsing! You are asking your own body to tell you what it likes and what it hates!

So this is our first real diet plan. I've been writing about it and teaching it for nearly 40 years. It's really a methodological approach, not a diet as such, designed to identify and eliminate specific foods which cause inflammation in your body.

You've probably heard of "anti-inflammatory foods" or such like. It's a sorry hoax perpetrated by very ignorant people.

The truth is there is no such thing as an anti-inflammatory food. Any food can be a problem and cause extensive inflammation; it's different in every single individual. For the same reason then, so-called "superfoods" are a folly and doctors like Stephen Pratt, who has made millions of dollars with his book, via Oprah Winfrey, has also condemned many people to be very sick. At least two of his "superfoods" are deadly for very many people: oats (in the grains/gluten family) and tomatoes (in the nightshade family).

I have had armies of people made seriously unwell by these two choices and several people made sick by every single "superfood" he mentions. It's a classic case of "experts" gaining knowledge by Googling for information, which is not based on direct clinical experience.

Food Addictions

Strangely, people often get addicted to their allergy foods. There is no need to explain to the reader the connection between being overweight and food addiction. But the allergy connection needs to be understood. The very foods that make a person ill are the ones consumed over and over, often on a daily basis. There is a reason for this, which 99.9% of doctors and health coaches don't even know: we call this effect hidden or "masked" food allergies.

What? Surely food allergies are obvious; the person eats the food, gets sick so he or she quits eating the food. How can it be "hidden" or unknown?

True, a person allergic to peanuts, strawberries or shellfish will know very quickly if they start eating the food. They consume it only occasionally and the severity of the reaction usually leaves no doubt about what is happening. It may even escalate to the point where the person begins to react dangerously to the allergen and may end up being rushed to ER, if he or she accidentally, or recklessly, consumes it.

That's not the kind of food allergy reaction I am talking about. Hidden allergies are the kind where the person is consuming a lot of that food, typically every day! This time there is no obvious reaction to pin-point the food. In fact symptoms may even start up on a day the person did not eat the food (withdrawal symptoms, if you like)!

Sure, this is getting ever more mysterious and hard to grasp. But bear with me and I'll explain this vital piece of slimming information in full.

If a person eats a food regularly, he or she may build up a reaction to the food. This is not a classical allergy, in the antigen-antibody sense, like for example hayfever or urticaria. It's more of an intolerance and is caused by repeated encounters with the food (basically overdosing on the food).

The fact is people tend to eat very repetitively, perhaps without realizing. Wheat, for example, is a food found in bread, cakes, biscuits, pastries, pizza, pasta, cookies, muffins and waffle batter, to name just a few foods—which are all the same thing, so far as the body is concerned! Indeed, I have been shocking patients for decades by telling them that bread and whisky are identical. Both contain wheat (or other grains) and yeast!

Corn shows up in almost all manufactured foods (they use it for cheap "padding"); caffeine is in many drinks, as you know; sugar is hidden in almost all manufactured foods; lettuce and tomato are common daily foods (salads!) but far from innocent.

So you need to start getting your head around the fact that our diets are extremely repetitious. Over-exposure is usually the start of the trouble and leads to the patient not being able to tolerate the food very well.

But it is rarely obvious. If you are allergic to dairy, you may not know it, because you consume milk on a daily basis (in tea, coffee, etc., even if you don't drink milk). Some days the symptoms are bad; some days not so bad. You may not make the connection between milk intake and your headaches, because you consume milk every day but don't get symptoms every day.

A person may even make the faulty logical step of saying, "I didn't have a single headache last week, but I drank milk every day. Therefore milk cannot be the problem." Oh yes it can! This is exactly why we call this effect the "hidden" food allergy.

The allergy could even be more deeply disguised, because the allergen *relieves* the symptom! It may be that the person gets a headache because he or she did NOT consume milk that day! This is where it gets interesting. But think about what you already know for a moment: *many people end up drinking coffee on an almost hourly basis, because if they didn't they would get the mother and father of a headache.* Dosing with coffee is keeping that headache away!

This is the origin of the term "masked" allergy. Repeated doses of the food masks or prevents the associated symptoms returning. If there is no intake of the specific food, then "withdrawal symptoms" come on.

By this stage you should be able to recognize all the effects of an addiction. Medically-speaking an addiction means there are associated withdrawal symptoms when the person tries to stop taking the drug in question. Why does a heroin addict keep injecting such a dangerous and costly substance? Because he or she feels better by doing so. The withdrawal symptoms are unpleasant but more heroin alleviates or "masks" those symptoms.

It's exactly the same mechanism with food!

Symptoms due to food addiction are very variable but are certainly not confined to just headaches and migraine. Low energy, joint pains, bellyaches, mood swings, depression, anxiety and of course over-eating, plus many other symptoms can have their basis in a hidden or "masked" food allergy.

In fact over-weight, under-weight and variable weight are classic markers for food allergy. Abdominal distress and bloating (that sudden expansion round the waistline) are also a giveaway.

Food binging, as it's known, is just a more extreme version of this whole masked allergy mechanism. The person tries to control their eating desires, until the withdrawal symptoms build up to the point where the body is screaming "Eat! Go for it!" And in the 1980s, incidentally, I was able to show it is the basis of serious eating disorders (anorexia and bulimia). Binging is NOT just about psychology and self-control.

The point is that, as well as causing unpleasant symptoms, an allergic food can also make you fat! I first found this out on the early 1980s when I began putting people on an exclusion (elimination) diet. Symptoms would typically lift but, regardless of that, patients routinely lost about 6 lbs. in the first week and then a very steady 2 lbs. a week thereafter.

It didn't seem to matter what the food allergies turned out to be. Even drinking black coffee (no milk, no sugar, no calories) can make you gain weight, if you are allergic to coffee! Undoubtedly, this is due to a water retention effect.

Hopefully, you will now have a fuller understanding of why individuals guzzle coffee after syrupy coffee, resulting in an intake of thousands of slurpy calories; or why someone would eat a whole bagful of cookies, after trying "just the one!" You may even recognize some of your own behavior in what I have just put before you!

This chapter is about how to expose and eradicate hidden food allergies. It's something that a careful and persistent individual can do, for him or herself. That's fortunate, because there are no reliable blood tests to detect food allergies. Your own body is the test bench. If you follow the instructions in the rest of this section, your body will tell you, loud and clear, what it likes and what it rejects!

When To Suspect A Food Allergy

There may be trouble with one or more foods when you experience any of the following symptoms (the more symptoms, the more certain it is you have a food allergy or intolerance).

- Bloating (can gain inches in a matter of minutes)
- Abdominal distress and flatulence (gas)
- Food binges
- Food cravings
- Diarrhea
- Constipation
- Variable bowel habit

- Symptoms actually come on while eating
- Symptoms after food (falling asleep, chills, sudden rapid heartbeat)
- Feeling unwell without food (food addiction)
- Feeling tired, crabby or very lethargic on waking (usually due to a withdrawal effect)

The last may seem strange: almost everybody wakes up feeling bad, don't they? True, but as I stated earlier, that's because almost everyone is suffering from food addictions!

Think about this: by the time we wake in the morning, we may not have eaten for 10 - 14 hours; that's more than enough time to set up withdrawal symptoms. With breakfast, we get our first "fix" of wheat, sugar, caffeine, or whatever the problem food is and the symptoms start to clear right away.

Particularly important are 5 key symptoms identified as being almost certain pointers to a food allergy:

- Overweight, underweight or wildly fluctuating weight (gain a few pounds in a day)
- Palpitations, unusually slow or rapid heartbeat, particularly after meals
- Excessive sweating, not related to exercise
- Persistent fatigue that isn't helped by rest
- Occasional swellings around the eyes, wrists, hands, abdomen or ankles

The characteristic of any allergy-related symptoms is that they come and go quickly; there one day, not there the next, back again a week later, and so on.

Secrets Of The Elimination Diet

The key to unlocking this troubling phenomenon is not just avoiding gluten and casein as the phoney "health researchers" on the internet will tell you. These two substances are only a fraction of the food allergens I have encountered over the years!

Commonly found food allergens include (not in any order) corn, sugar, tea, coffee, orange, potato and egg. In truth, any food can become an allergen, especially if you over-indulge it. Be warned.

The key to solving the difficulty is the clever use of an elimination diet (sometime called an exclusion diet). The trick is to avoid all the likely troublemakers at once. This is because of what we call the "eight nails in the shoe" trap: if you have eight nails sticking up in your shoe, you will limp with pain. But if you pull out just one of these nails, you'll still limp!

If you give up one test food at a time, you may see no improvement, because there are several other food allergens (quite commonly so).

So we use a more comprehensive elimination diet: the "Stone Age diet" which, yes, is the origin of the modern paleo eating principle. It just so happens that the commonest food allergens are the unnatural foods which our caveman ancestors did not eat: grains, dairy, tea, coffee, sugar, alcohol, and of course our ubiquitous manufactured foods. These are what I call farmer foods, since we have only eaten these items since we ceased our nomadic existence and settled the land.

Our ancestors would have eaten a hunter-gatherer diet. That means eating foods that could be obtained by walking through forests and over plains: meat, fish, fruit, berries, roots, leaves (vegetables) and drinking only water.

So we eat like cavemen for a week or two and see what happens as a result. Now here is a very important principle: this is a test diet, not a maintenance diet. We use it to work out any foods that are not suiting you. So even if you feel really good on the Stone Age diet, don't just stick with it: you must follow through, to find out which were the actual culprit foods.

If you give up twenty foods, lose weight fast and feel tons better, it does not mean all twenty foods were the problem. It may only have been one, or two, or three items. You need to know which are the enemy foods.

We establish which ones cause trouble using what we call "food challenge testing". That's when we ask your body, "Do you tolerate this food, or not?" Do it right and you will find it's easy to get reliable answers.

The Stone Age Exclusion Diet

You must strictly give up the banned foods; not eat even a forkful, otherwise you might miss the results. We are trying to completely eliminate suspect foods from your body. The whole reason a food allergy can hide is because of food residues in your bowel. It takes about four days for food to transit your bowel, so if you eat the food twice or more in a week, there is always some inside you!

So when you eat some more, nothing may happen! The challenge test would fail! Sometimes there could be immediate symptoms but often not. That's how it gets missed. To succeed we have to completely clear your bowel of the suspect foods.

But if you cheat, even just a tiny bit, it puts more of the food in your gut, resets the counter back to zero, and the four days clearance starts all over again. Don't do it.

And this is where understanding adulterated foods is important. Manufactured foods may contain repetitious amounts of several foods. If you nibble a bit of bread one day and then take a forkful of pasta a few days later, you are repeatedly exposing your body to wheat, the principle ingredient of both foods.

OK, shocking enough; but no big surprise to most of us, really. We know that junk food isn't good for us (hence the name) and obesity is just one of the many negatives arising from the consumption of manufactured food items.

But now what may be a REAL shock to most people. Unadulterated whole foods—yes, even organic whole foods—can still make you ill.

Everyone thinks of the negatives of processed food. But that's not what food allergies are all about. Even good foods can make you sick, if you don't tolerate them well or are allergic to them. I have had patients made seriously ill with any food you can name: epilepsy due to carrots, colitis due to lettuce, eczema due to potato, and asthma due to tomatoes are four examples among tens of thousands of cases known to me.

So there is a lot to be gained by sifting through your diet, to see if any foodstuffs disagree with you. Remember... food addiction is one of the main symptoms of food allergy and nobody needs to have the connection between food addiction and overweight spelled out!

There is a happy bonus. You may find you shed the pounds and, at the same time, get rid of your headache, asthma, eczema, arthritis, colitis or whatever.

It's a journey of discovery I believe everyone should undertake, at least once in their lifetime!

Here's A Simple Summary Of The Stone Age Diet

Foods You Are Not Allowed To Eat:

- No stimulant drinks – no tea, coffee, alcohol
- No sugar, honey, additives or sweeteners
- No grains: absolutely no wheat, corn, rye, rice, barley, oats or millet. That means no bread, cakes, muffins, biscuits, granola, pastry, flour or farina.
- No milk or dairy produce: no skimmed milk, cream, butter, margarines or spreads, not even goat's milk
- No eggs and preferably no chicken (same animal!)
- No citrus foods
- No manufactured food: nothing from tins, packets, bottles or jars. The safe rule is: If somebody labeled it, they likely added to it.

So what's left? Hundreds of foods! Real foods, tasty foods!

Foods You Are Allowed To Eat:

- Any fresh, whole meat or offal (not processed or smoked)
- Any vegetables (fresh or frozen, not tinned)
- Any fruit, except the citrus family (no orange, lime, lemon etc.)
- Any fish (not processed or smoked)
- Quinoa and buckwheat (grain substitutes but beware nobody has mixed these with wheat flour)
- All fresh unsweetened fruit juices are allowed, except citrus
- Nuts (any except candied or coated in any way)
- Herb teas (careful: some contain citrus peel)
- Spring water, preferably bottled in glass
- Fresh whole herbs
- Salt and pepper to taste

Don't forget about addictions. It is quite likely that you will get withdrawal symptoms during the first few days excluding foods. This is actually good news because it means you have given up something important! Usually the effects are mild and amount to nothing more than feeling irritable, tired, or perhaps having a headache, but be warned—it could put you in bed for a couple of days. I have seen wheat "cold turkey" that was just as grim as getting off narcotics.

Please also note that it is possible to be allergic even to the allowed foods; they are chosen simply because reactions to them are less common. If you are in this minority, you might temporarily feel worse on this diet, but at least it proves you have a food allergy. In that case, try eliminating the foods you are eating more of (potato is a common offender; giving up meat might work) and see if you then begin to improve.

If not, you could consider eating only lamb and pears for 4 – 5 days, an allergy hack which I call a "half fast". The two foods are chosen because they are relatively rare food allergens. Then proceed to food challenge testing, as below.

Patients sometimes ask: *What about my vitamin and mineral supplements while on an elimination diet, can I keep taking those?* The answer is: best not to. Most vitamin and mineral tablets contain hidden food ingredients, such as corn starch. Even those that say "allergy-free" formulas are misleading. They may not be made up with common allergens, such as wheat, corn or soya derivatives; but nevertheless, vegetable ingredients are present, such as rice polishings and potato starch. To call these "allergy safe" or even hypoallergenic is, in my view, dishonest.

Don't take the risk, because you won't come to any harm without supplements for a few days.

Integrating this approach with other regimens, like keto and paleo (see section 14). They are fully compatible. My advice is just concentrate on one thing at once: find and eliminate your food allergens and then do keto or paleo separately. The important point to bear in mind is that, to unmask hidden food allergies, you must strictly avoid the food for a few days. Cheating or cutting corners may deny you the valuable information you need.

Food Challenge Testing

After the four-day unmasking period has elapsed (longer if you have been constipated), you can begin challenge testing.

Now is the time to test each food meticulously, to see if it might cause symptoms. It is not enough to feel well on a very restricted diet; we want to know *why?* Which are the real culprits? These are the foods you must avoid long-term, not all those which are banned at the beginning.

Even if you don't feel well, as already pointed out, this does not prove you have no allergies amongst the foods you gave up. Test the foods as you re-introduce them, anyway; you may be in for a surprise.

FORGET THE DOGMA: you are unique. So we are not interested in crusader ideas or dogma, such as veganism, vegetarianism, "The Maker's Diet" or lectin theory. Every single set diet will make some individuals ill, even if it helps others. I repeat this important message over and over in this book, and now you know why!

My recommended testing procedure is as follows:

1. Eat a substantial helping of the food, preferably on its own for the first exposure. Lunch is the ideal meal for this.

2. Choose only whole, single foods, not mixtures and recipes. Try to get supplies that have not been chemically treated in any way.

3. Wait several hours to see if there is an immediate reaction, and if not, eat some more of the food, along with a typical ordinary evening meal.

4. You may eat a third, or fourth, portion if you want, to be sure.

5. Take your resting pulse (sit still for two minutes) before, and several times during, the first 90 minutes after the first exposure to the food. These days it is easy to get a pulse reading, with the ubiquitous smartphone health monitors and related apps. A rise of ten or more beats in the RESTING pulse is a fairly reliable sign of an allergy. However, no change in the pulse does **not** mean the food is safe, unless symptoms are absent also.

If you do experience an unpleasant reaction, take Epsom salts. Also, alkali salts (a mixture of two parts sodium bicarbonate to one part potassium bicarbonate: one teaspoonful in a few ounces of lukewarm water) should help. Discontinue further tests until symptoms have abated once more. This is very important, as you cannot properly test when symptoms are already present; you are looking for foods which trigger symptoms.

Using the above approach, you should be able to reliably test one food a day, minimum. Go rapidly if all is well, because the longer you stay off a food, the more the allergy (if there is one) will tend to die down and you may miss it.

Occasionally, patients experience a 'build up' which causes confusion and sometimes failure. Suspect this if you felt better on the exclusion diet, but you gradually became ill again when re-introducing foods, and can't really say why. Perhaps there were no noticeable reactions.

In that case, eliminate all the foods you have re-introduced until your symptoms clear again, then re-introduce them more slowly. This time, eat the foods steadily, several times a day for three to four days before making up your mind. It is unlikely that one will slip the net with this approach.

Once you have accepted a food as safe, of course you must avoid eating it frequently, otherwise it too may become an allergy. Eat it once a day at most - only every four days when you have enough 'safe' foods to accomplish this.

Use Weighings To Detect Problems

You can use your weight as a monitor in food challenge testing. Weigh yourself before challenging a food and again 6 – 8 hours later. If you find yourself putting on surprise pounds, suspect the newly introduced food may be the problem. It could have caused inflammation and made you retain water.

This additional clue can be valuable and is important, even in the absence of actual symptoms of feeling unwell.

Keto Monitor

Later, you'll learn the magic of keto dieting and how to monitor it, using a ketone/blood glucose meter. It will show you if anything throws off your weight-control strategy, resulting in a surge of blood glucose.

What we've learned is that certain foods will spike blood glucose or lower keto status and this denotes just another type of food intolerance. With patience and proper usage of your keto meter (I have the KetoMojo device), you can track down foods that cause an unwanted glucose spike about an hour after a meal and avoid them, just as if the food gave you a headache or a rash!

Note that "keto friendly" foods, such as cabbage, cheese and bullet-proof coffee can cause a spike in blood sugar. So this is an important extra detection method. It will help you get in the zone!

On my *Eternity Health and Happiness* program, you will actually be given a wearable blood glucose monitor for a couple of weeks. It can reveal astonishing food reactions that are not healthy and yet you didn't know you had! (www.healthandhappiness.com)

Your Personal Exclusion Program

Once you have carried out the challenge tests you will have a list of items which you are intolerant of, or which cause you to gain weight. You must now avoid these, if you are serious about your health. You have, in effect, designed your own personal diet plan for life. Use it as something you return to in times of trouble or stress, a safe platform to fall back on.

There should be no rush to try and re-introduce any of the rogue items, if at all. Design your living and eating plan without them, long-term. However the good news is that allergies do settle down, sometimes quite rapidly. If you develop and practice a newer safer ecological lifestyle, you may have surprisingly little further trouble. You may feel better than you have felt in years and the excess weight comes tumbling off!

Many patients feel and act younger, so much so that friends and relatives often comment. I noticed this over thirty years ago and that is one of the reasons I now find myself part of the anti-aging movement.

Some Questions

The exclusion diet worked well but once I had tested and re-introduced all the foods, I went back to having symptoms. Why?

The fact that you did feel better means that for sure you did have food allergies. But you failed to detect them with your challenge testing and so allowed unsafe foods back in your diet. There is little choice but to go over the ground once again: re-start the full exclusion diet for a few days, until symptoms re-clear and then re-test all the foods, going more slowly. This time have maybe 2 days of steady eating on each new food, before you pronounce it safe.

Alternatively, you may opt to go straight for allergy testing. Blood test panels are not very reliable. IgE testing only picks up the most extreme type of allergy or intolerance. Skin prick and scratch tests are almost worthless for food reactions.

I would rather recommend intradermal testing by Miller's method (also known as provocation-neutralization testing) is a fast alternative. In just a few hours you can find out what weeks of dieting and challenge may miss. Not only that but you can get an "antidote" formula, which will help.

In no circumstances would I suggest orthodox allergy "desensitization" injections. Nor should any doctors offer it to you, since it has been pronounced dangerous by all doctors who do not make money by doing it!

I was doing great until I had a virus. Since then all my symptoms are back. Can an infection really do this?

It certainly can. If your immune system goes under stress, because of a bacterial or virus invader, the crisis can trigger the emergence of many allergies, old and new. I usually tell patients to go back on the exclusion program for a few days, until the crisis is past, then go back to your personal food plan. If you are using Miller's end-point vaccines, just described, you may possibly need to have these retuned by your physician.

If you need more detailed help, I have written a comprehensive self-help guide, called *Diet Wise*. You can get a copy here: www.dietwisebook.com

Quenching The Gut Fire

To learn more about quenching gut fire and turning off bad genes, get yourself a copy of *Diet Wise* and go over to the Diet Wise Academy and watch some free explanatory videos.

www.dietwiseacademy.com

You can sign up at the academy, if you need more advanced help.

You may also find my *Fire In The Belly* book fills in a lot of blanks!

www.fireinthebellybook.com

A Note About Cytotoxic Blood Testing

You may learn about blood testing for allergies. Let me fill you in. Conventional blood tests measure immune parameters, like IgA and IgE (Elisa tests). These are accurate only for the extreme type-1 hypersensitivity to food, not the masked allergy mechanism I have been talking about. Type 1 hypersensitivity is the kind that produces rapid and sometimes fatal reactions to peanuts and other foods but is very rare. If you have the problem, you'll know about it. These pages are not for you.

There is another kind of laboratory test called cytotoxic testing (example: the ALCAT test). A person's blood is exposed to a panel of food allergens and, depending on which ones damage the white blood cells (hence the term cytotoxic), an allergy is diagnosed.

You'll hear and see many wonderful claims for this approach. But you need to be cautious. Most of the marketing of this system depends heavily on "testimonials" or endorsements, which means that science is rather lacking. True some people do well and get a good outcome. But many waste their money and of course you are not told about this by those peddling the method.

Cytotoxic testing is troubled by many false negatives. Being told you have an allergy to a food when you don't (a false positive) it not really a problem. You avoid the food anyway, that's it. But a false negative—being told you are not allergic to a food, when in fact you are—is likely to stall any further progress. You innocently eat the food and it causes problems but you are firmly of the belief that this food is not an issue.

There is an improvement on the original cytotoxic testing method called LEAP testing (lifestyle, eating and performance). It may be more accurate because it measures volumetric change (damage) in cells, as opposed to the normal two-dimensional counting method under a microscope. Much is boasted for this test and clearly most of the claims are marketing in nature, rather than science-based.

It is often coupled with the MRT® test, patented and belonging to Oxford Biomedical Technologies Inc., Riviera Beach, Florida (it's funny how some companies use the word "Oxford" to try and attract extra credibility, by implying some connection with the venerable old UK city of the same name).

MRT stands for Mediator Release Testing, which measures inflammatory mediator levels as a result of food sensitivities. All food reactions involve cytokine mediator release, which is responsible for the inflammatory surges, seen as a result of eating an offending food. Mediator release provokes volumetric changes (swelling) in neutrophils, monocytes, eosinophils, and lymphocytes.

Americans seem to think that something being patented means the same as scientifically validated which, of course, it does not. Perhaps that's why they push hard on the point that their test has been patented. It sells!

You can find Oxford Biomedical Technologies Inc. here (far away from Oxford):

3555 Fiscal Court
Suites 8 & 9,
Riviera Beach, FL 33404
Phone: (888) 669-5327, (561) 848-7111
Website: https://nowleap.com

PART 2. THE ISSUES

SECTION 6.
METABOLIC SYNDROME AND DIABESITY

There has been lots of speculation about why we have an "epidemic" of obesity today. Favorite among knowledgeable doctors and nutritionists is definitely the inclusion of too much carbohydrate in government dietary recommendations, such as the now-discredited former US government "Food Pyramid".

What do farmers use to fatten up their livestock; make them fat and heavy, so they get more profits?

Carbohydrates.

What's the one class of foods that causes addictions and cravings? Fat? No. Proteins? No.

Carbohydrates.

What class of foods so disorders insulin control of blood sugar that the body stops reacting to healthy signals, leading to the deposit of excess fat?

Carbohydrates.

Are you getting the picture? There is no question that government "expert" insistence that we all need up to 65% of carbohydrate in our diet to be healthy is criminally stupid. Feeding that stuff to kids is madness and sets them up for a lifetime of struggle against weight issues.

The results are clear: the rise in obesity statistics have almost exactly paralleled the inclusion of more and more carbohydrate in our standard diet—especially refined carbohydrates, such as white sugar, white flour, potato fries and sugar syrup (HCFS).

Today, in the US alone, there is not one state with less than 20% of the population obese. That varies from Colorado (20.5%) to Louisiana (34.7%). Obesity, for this league table, is defined as a body mass index (BMI) of more than 30. (That translates to more than 197 pounds on a 5'8" person).

Europe is slightly better but not good.

Diabesity: More Than A Joke

Obesity and diabetes are so closely interconnected that one wit coined the term "diabesity" for a new health condition that's prevalent today. The term is now a trademark owned by Shape Up America, itself founded in 1994 by former US Surgeon General C. Everett Koop to raise awareness of the dangerous health effects of obesity.

It's a great aide memoire but I am going to work with the more scientific term: "the metabolic syndrome".

Originally known as "syndrome X', because no-one knew the cause, this condition was first described and named by Gerald Reaven MD, an American endocrinologist and professor emeritus in medicine at the Stanford University School Of Medicine.

The principle criteria for metabolic syndrome are: high blood pressure, obesity (central belly fat), high blood sugar, insulin resistance, high triglycerides and low HDL (or good) cholesterol. It increases the risk of diabetes, heart disease and death.

It's time to get real about this issue. Obesity is dangerous: it shortens your life. Insurance actuaries load premiums according to an individual's weight. Why? The reason is simple and prep-school math standard: the more overweight you are, the shorter your life, in statistical terms.

Of course some people beat the odds but if you look at the increasing army of centenarians (those aged over 100 years), none of them are even fat, never mind obese. Nuff said?

A 2009 study funded mainly by the UK Medical Research Council, the British Heart Foundation, Cancer Research UK, the EU BIOMED programme and the US National Institute on Aging, found that:

People who are obese could reduce their lifespan by three years.

People who are overweight but not obese—with a Body Mass Index (BMI) between 25 and 29.9—could shorten their lifespans by a year.

Extreme obesity—weighing 100 pounds or more above a healthy weight—is as bad for your health as a lifelong smoking habit, shortening your lifespan by as much as 10 years.

Above a healthy weight, every 5-point jump in BMI increases your risk of early death by roughly 30 percent.

Researchers reviewed 57 studies, which tracked the health of some 900,000 adults for 10 to 15 years, and analyzed about 70,000 deaths. That's a MASSIVE study. Their findings were reported online and in The Lancet.[1]

Doctors continue to argue over the finer details but the big picture is simple: you cannot be seriously overweight and "healthy". Your blood pressure, blood fats and blood control will go to hell, for a start. Diabetes is almost a certainty. Sudden death very much on the cards.

So if looking good doesn't motivate you to deal with serious weight issues, then avoidance of early death should.

And if you already have diabetes and are taking medication, don't be smug. Let me give you the bad news: taking diabetes-control drugs has not been shown to increase lifespan back towards normal. And, worse still, even keeping blood sugar levels accurately within recommended bounds does not save your life, nor prevent the relentless organ damage that comes with diabetes.

You are going to die sooner, on average, unless you shed that weight and control those dangerous fat-packing carbs.

Stepping back, diabetes is an autoimmune and highly inflammatory condition. You need to reduce inflammation in your tissues. Fat, especially belly fat, is highly inflammatory.

Dangerous "Belly Fat"

The Greek physician Hippocrates was on to this nearly 2500 years ago! He observed that, "Sudden death is more common in those who are naturally fat than in the lean," (400 BC). For many centuries, this astute observation went completely unexplained and was eventually ignored.

While people in the 20th century have been persuaded to worry about fats in the blood, such as cholesterol and triglycerides, it has turned out that Hippocrates was right. Body fat, especially central belly fat, is the real cause of the problems leading to heart disease.

How could that be? Surely blood fats are what cause blockage in our arteries, leading to coronary artery obstruction?

In fact that is not so. We have learned that inflammation is what blocks arteries; so much so that sudden death is more commonly attributable to clotting caused by inflammatory lesions in the blood vessels, than what is supposed to be actual silting up of arteries with fat. In other words, the narrowed portions of the coronary arteries are not always where the fatal clots tend to occur but wide open sections, where inflammation is taking place.

Still not enough to fully make sense, is it? But if you add to all this the fact that belly flat is highly inflammatory in nature, the new and more accurate model of heart disease becomes easily understandable. It means the association between obesity, fatty arteries, inflammation and heart disease is still valid but the mechanism is more complicated than we thought.

The new view explains certain mysteries; like why an obese person could live a full life, even though statistical odds are against him or her (little inflammation) and why a young, not overweight, fit individual might drop dead suddenly, early in life (inflammatory markers high).

Inflammation has emerged as the true killer. But belly fat has also emerged as one of the main sources of dangerous systemic inflammation, as we shall see. So you need to get rid of those extra pounds round the waist, before they get rid of you!

Explaining Belly Fat

Everyone has some fatty tissue on board, called adipose tissue. Mostly it is found just under the skin in the thighs, hips, buttocks, and abdomen and is called subcutaneous fat. Before the menopause, subcutaneous fat gives women their cute, sexy proportions that men like. But excess diet-induced weight gain causes a rise in so-called visceral fat: fat surrounding our internal organs (heart, lungs, digestive tract, liver, etc.) in the chest, abdomen, and pelvis. Men under 40 tend to have a higher proportion of visceral fat to subcutaneous fat than women. But women start to store more visceral fat after the menopause.

Belly fat is just the visible protrusion of this visceral fat.

What is sinister is that up to 60% of all cells found in excess visceral fat are macrophages, whereas subcutaneous fat is populated with only 5% to 10% macrophages. Macrophages are sure markers for inflammation, so this accumulation in belly fat spells big trouble. [2]

No question: *visceral fat causes inflammation and is dangerous, by its very nature.*

There is no way to selectively reduce visible belly fat. You need to get rid of all excess fat and thus it will come off your belly at the same time. Tips for working your abs and flattening them are misguided. If you have understood the dangers of visceral fat written about here, you wouldn't want to simply disguise its presence, would you?

As well as heart disease and diabetes, visceral fat plays a role in aging and even cancer formation.

Get rid of it!

Eliminating Metabolic Syndrome

Surprisingly, metabolic syndrome is very easy to control and eliminate. You don't really need medications, like Metformin and blood pressure drugs. All it takes is a simple change in diet and lifestyle. Conventional doctors do not manage this deadly condition well, because they've got the wrong cause in their heads. They believe it's all down to saturated fat and cholesterol in the diet. The true cause is excess carbohydrates.

So the most important counter-remedy is to eliminate most or all carbohydrates, especially refined carbs, such as sugar, white flour and corn sugar (HFCS). Make an effort to give up grains (plants from the grass family, such as wheat, corn, rye, oats, rice). Effectively, that means giving up all manufactured foods (refer to section 3).

Instead, eat a diet close to the ancestral hunter-gatherers diet. IGNORE THE VEGETARIANS AND VEGANS: you cannot eat grains from any source if you have metabolic syndrome and vegetarians tend to rely heavily on grains. You need to give up milk too. Milk is a sugar food (lactose), so skimmed milk, far from being healthy, is actually worse for you, because the sugar is even more concentrated. You'd do better to keep the butter and cream and toss the skimmed!

Instead, fill up on meat, fowl and fish, with vegetables, salads and fruit, much as our caveman ancestors ate. Before humans over-hunted animals and turned to plant sources of foods, they were superbly tall and healthy, as testified by their perfect skeletons. But after switching to more vegetables and plants, arthritis appeared and Humankind began to shrink.

Only in the latter part of the 20th century did we grow back to our prehistoric average height. This is from pure archeological evidence, by the way, not theories and dogma.

Add in healthy saturated fat to your diet: cream, egg yolks, cheese, coconut oil and these will help you lose weight quickly, partly by reducing your appetite and partly by switching your body's metabolic processes to turn off the "fat switch".

The what?

Yes, there really is a switch you can flip to on or off! On, you pile on the fat; off, you lose weight quickly and easily. This is more stunning new science and great news for the slimmer who is struggling.

The Fat Switch

It's a metaphor for the idea that creating fat in our bodies can be turned on, or turned off. How marvelous it would be to flip the switch to *off* and start burning fat, instead of accumulating fat!

Well, we've arrived at that point, thanks to the pioneer work of experts like professor Richard J. Johnson, at the University of Colorado, Denver. Johnson has published several papers which are quite pivotal in our understanding of why we accumulate fat and why that has been driven to happen so much in the last 50 years or so.

Johnson wanted to understand the exact mechanism. Instead of walking the orthodox path, and using limited orthodox thinking (biochemistry, genetics, cellular pathology) he decided to tackle it from a much broader perspective: history, epidemiology, anthropology, paleontology and evolutionary science.

He asked himself and his team why it was that some animals go through periods of rapid fat gain and then could somehow switch to a fat-burning mode. A hibernating bear, for example, could gain hundreds of pounds in the Fall and get fat for hibernation. But then it would switch to fat-burning mode and live off it's fat deposits while sleeping for the whole winter. The fat gain mode exactly parallels the human "disease" we call metabolic syndrome (or diabesity), even including fatty liver deposits.

The tiny humming bird, incredibly, follows the same cycle. During the day humming birds feed frenetically, and pile on fat, so much so that their little livers turn creamy white with fat deposits. But then they go through night unable to eat but living off the day's fat deposits, which vanish by sunrise and the whole cycle starts all over again.

So maybe what we call "metabolic syndrome" is just a natural process. It seems that nature uses it often. But since we can't understand it or control it, then for us it is a danger, the equivalent of a disease. We don't hibernate but maybe we are doing something that triggers the fat storage mode, just as if we were intending to hibernate?

Well, suffice it to say that this entirely fresh way of looking at the problem has revealed some amazingly valuable answers. We now know there is a fat switch and how it works. Moreover, we know how to turn it off! Are you ready?

The AMP Pathway

The secret lies in a funny molecule called adenosine monophosphate (AMP) and its fate within the body. AMP is an energy molecule, obviously related to ATP (adenosine triphosphate) our main energy-bearing molecule.

In the process of metabolism of sugars (glucose) to create energy, AMP can be transformed by one of two enzymes, according to whichever "wins". AMP deaminase (AMPD) leads to fat accumulation. AMP kinase (AMPK) leads to fat burning. In other words AMPK determines our body fat composition and especially the amount of visceral "belly" fat that we carry. Its activity is also tied to our life expectancy. When we are young, AMPK is more active, but as we age, the cellular AMPK activation decreases, leading to visceral fat accumulation and loss of muscle mass.

So there is the switch: AMPD we deposit unwanted fat; AMPK, we burn fat and get slim. Hooray for AMPK!

We get AMPD or AMPK—one or the other—according to influencing factors. Insulin resistance, for example, is associated with lack of AMPK and excess AMPD. We need insulin to metabolize excess glucose safely. If the body stops responding to insulin (insulin resistance), then the excess sugars in the diet convert automatically to unwanted fat.

That's exactly what happens when we start to consume large quantities of sugar or carbs (most carbs convert readily to sugars). The healthy pathway is overloaded and breaks down. Instead of our mitochondria being able to process normal glucose quantities to ATP, they switch to fat depositing mode.

But it gets worse: AMPD also leads to leptin resistance. Leptin is a so-called "hunger hormone" and it switches off the feeling of wanting to eat. Its opposite number is another hunger hormone called ghrelin, which makes you feel peckish! (see section 4 to read more about hunger hormones) Readers will readily see that leptin is the one we want! It lessens our appetite. But if leptin resistance sets in, the body stops listening. In other words, eating will still trigger leptin release but it's ignored. You go on eating anyway, eating a LOT!

Leptin resistance is crucial to overeating and gluttony.

All this is reversed by generating AMPK, which displaces AMPD. Where do we get AMPK? There are con-artists selling it on Amazon already, as if all you had to do was swallow a few capsules and disregard your lifestyle. Not true.

But there are important natural ways to ramp up AMPK. Changing how you eat is the most important. Intermittent fasting is the way to go. Keto dieting, the current craze, is effective too. More of that in a later section.

Herbs

The following herb substances inhibit AMPD and stimulate AMPK:

- Berberine. Berberine works just as well as metformin, the main diabetes medication used by doctors.

- Gynostemma. Gynostemma works twice as well as metoformin for weight loss and diabetes control!

- Quercetin is a plant flavonol that helps increase AMPK levels. It also increases insulin sensitivity

- Acetyl-L-Carnitine (ALCAR), another substance that lowers AMPD and increases AMPK levels. It helps lower insulin resistance as well as being a powerful antioxidant. It is known as a neuro-protective and neurogenerative compound. I have given you generous quantities of acetyl-L-carnitine in my Mito-Cell Rejuvenator: (https://drkeithsown.com/mito-cell/)

Now you know why!

The Fructose Story

To get to the heart of this fat switch issue, you need to understand the role of fructose. Remember table sugar (sucrose) is 50% glucose and 50% fructose. It's "natural".

But what is far from natural is the HUGE quantity of sugar we now consume. It's gone up to an average of over 130 lbs. per person per year in Western countries (and those that follow us, like India). Not just added sugar, but hidden sugar, in foods such as bread, ketchup, ham, cereals and yoghurt. That means we swallow HUGE quantities of fructose and that in turn means trouble.

Add to that the fact that the food industry has been corrupting soft drinks and juices in particular with MEGA-quantities of concentrated fructose, in the form of high-fructose corn syrup (HFCS).

Put these two together and you can say that we consume hundreds of times more fructose now than even the recent past (say 70 years ago).

Unfortunately, fructose completely blocks the mechanism of the fat OFF switch. It does this by leading to excess of AMPD and it seriously inhibits AMPK.

YOU CANNOT AFFORD TO EAT FRUCTOSE (though curiously enough, Prof. Johnson has conducted trials and concluded that eating natural fruits in moderation does not upset the fat switch!)

In fact you cannot afford to eat any sugar. We have way too much of it and the incidence of obesity and diabetes exactly parallels the quantities of sugar in our diets (see graphs):

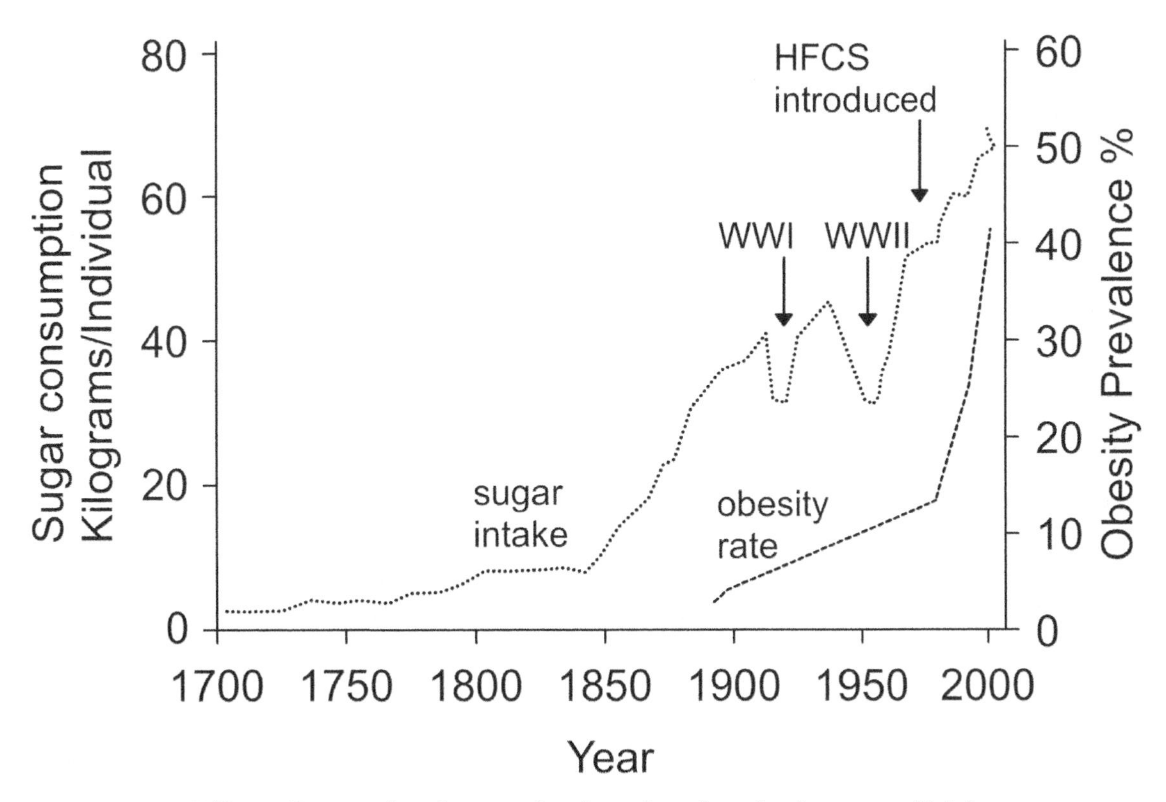

Effect of sugar intake on obesity, showing the impact of high fructose corn syrup (HFCS)

Just give up adding sugar and avoid foods where it is hidden and you will do very well. Your palate will adjust very quickly and within a couple of weeks at most you won't even notice it's gone from your diet!

Help your mitochondria to help you lose weight or maintain a healthy weight. They know what to do! Just don't flood them with junk sugar that's put there solely to get you addicted to manufactured food products.

Beer: unfortunately, beer also promotes AMPD and lowers AMPK. Wine and champagne are far safer, as I have been broadcasting for YEARS.

Uric Acid

There is another twist to the story, which gives us a surprising biomarker, to tell how healthy our metabolism is; that's uric acid. It is a marker for the AMPD pathway (therefore raised levels are bad).

The appearance of uric acid means something is wrong. Uric acid comes from the breakdown of DNA, RNA and ATP. These three health molecules are crucial and should not be damaged in any significant way.

In fact animals in the wild seem to get very agitated and disturbed when uric acid levels rise in their blood. Prof. Johnson reasons that this is because matters have progressed beyond glycogen and fat consumption and the body is beginning to “consume” its own muscles, to provide energy.

Without knowing any physiology or biochemistry, the animal just knows it’s an emergency and to get busy finding food, quickly. In fact the emperor penguin—nature’s most impeccable father—will lose heart and abandon the egg he is nurturing and head for the sea, to find fresh food. That’s how strong the uric acid signal is!

We can learn from this.

Uric acid should be on any blood test panel for someone overweight. It tells us which way the fat switch is set. That’s very valuable knowledge, as you will now understand.

PART 2. THE ISSUES

SECTION 7. INFLAMMATION IS CRUCIAL

Belly Fat Is Proven Inflammatory

The trouble is fat doesn't just sit idle; it acts like an organ and secretes inflammatory substances called adipokines. Also it holds onto fat-soluble toxic compounds like pesticides and other pollutants and can release them over time. Those too have an inflammatory effect.

The earliest indication that fats act this way was a 1985 report, noting positive correlations between body mass and the peripheral leukocyte count (the latter is a marker for inflammation). [1]

Since then, a large number of studies have found that increased body mass index (BMI) correlates with increases in systemic circulating levels of a whole host of inflammatory proteins, including ones you may know: C-Reactive Protein (CRP), Interleukin-6 (IL-6), vascular cell adhesion molecule 1 (VCAM-1), fibrinogen and angiotensinogen. Considering that adipose tissue and adipocytes produce all of these factors, it can be inferred that adipose tissue itself is a large contributor to many systemic diseases. [2]

The matter was put beyond doubt when an Italian surgical team decided to measure the inflammatory markers in the portal veins of their subjects. The portal vein is filled with blood that drains visceral fat, and in this study was shown to have very high levels of IL-6, a notorious inflammatory cytokine. Increased IL-6 levels in the portal vein correlated with concentrations of C-reactive protein (CRP) in the body, which is one of our most important markers for inflammation, and chronic inflammation is in turn directly associated with insulin resistance, hypertension, type 2 diabetes and atherosclerosis, among other things. [3]

There is at least one other important mechanism by which fats harm us. Unfortunately, in an obese person, the body can run out of safe places to store fat and begin storing it in and around the vital organs, such as the heart and the liver.

Non-alcoholic fatty liver disease (NAFLD) was once rare. But with obesity increasing, it occurs more and more. In this condition, the liver is damaged by deposits of fats throughout the organ, strangling its normal functions. Liver damage can eventually lead to a fibrosis process called cirrhosis. NAFLD causes more cirrhosis than alcohol abuse (over half of all cirrhosis cases are due to NAFLD, compared to 6% caused by alcohol abuse), so this is a critical subject. Let me repeat: *obesity leads to far more liver damage and cirrhosis than alcoholism.*

NAFLD and metabolic syndrome go hand in hand. NAFLD has now reached epidemic portions. In the USA alone the incidence is between 80 and 100 million individuals. Many patients don't even know they have it. The majority of the patients are obese but the disease can affect non-obese individuals as well. Although the disease remains asymptomatic most of the time, it can slowly progress to end stage liver disease. It will be the most common indication of liver transplantation in the [4]future.

You Have To Work It Off

Unfortunately, studies make it very clear that you have to lose the fat legitimately, to benefit your health. Liposuction, for instance, does no good. It may reduce your weight and waistline temporarily but it only removes subcutaneous fat, not dangerous visceral fat. Don't waste your money.

An important study reported in the June 17 issue of *The New England Journal of Medicine*, showed that removing large amounts of subcutaneous fat from beneath the skin—about 20% of a person's total body fat mass—brought no beneficial medical effects in terms of reduced inflammation. These results demonstrate that decreasing fat mass by surgery, which removes billions of fat cells, does not actually provide the metabolic benefits seen when fat mass is reduced by dietary changes.

Doing it the right way shrinks the size of fat cells and decreases the amount of fat inside the abdomen and other tissues, as well as subcutaneous fat. [5]

You are holding the right source book in your hand for reducing belly fat. You must lose weight and choose, among the many strategies given here, one which will give you maximum satisfaction in slimming and keeping the weight off permanently.

The Role Of Omega 7

No, it's not a typo. You've heard of omega-6s (bad) and omega-3s (good). But omega-7 is a new name in the game. Even as I write, Harvard is scrabbling to try and patent this natural fatty acid.

"Fatty acids" are essential to human life because they are the cell's primary energy source. Fatty acids also serve as cellular structural components.

Ingesting the proper fatty acids confers significant health and longevity benefits, including weight control. Over weight is characterized by inflammation and the right fatty acids quench inflammation. This is entirely consistent with my platform here, which is that you MUST beat inflammation, in order to successfully lose weight.

The typical American diet contains plenty of omega-6s, but is woefully deficient in omega-3s and monounsaturated fats. This makes systemic inflammation almost inevitable. Thus there is a consensus to eat more foods rich in omega-3s (fish and some nuts) and monounsaturated fats (from olive oil and some nuts). Coconut oil, too, is a very serious health player in this field and leads to numerous benefits, apart from weight loss, despite a crackpot "professor" from Harvard University pronouncing it to be a true "poison".

But now there is a new kid on the block.

Scientists at Harvard Medical School and the Cleveland Clinic have been investigating a novel fatty acid called omega-7 (palmitoleic acid), which can help break the cycle of high blood sugar, elevated lipid levels, inflammation, and excess fat gain as well as enhance insulin sensitivity.[6]

Omega-7 has been shown to cause an increase in fat breakdown and an increase in the enzymes involved in fat burning for energy. Additionally, omega-7 can reduce new fat synthesis in the body, so that helps you not to pile weight back on.

Researchers have found that by taking omega-7 for just 30 days, patients had a 44% reduction in C-reactive protein (important measure of inflammation) levels. That's massive and way beyond anything that can be achieved by conventional anti-inflammatory treatments.[7]

In yet another study, involving 3,630 American men and women, researchers also found that higher levels of omega-7 were strongly associated with numerous positive health factors. This includes lower LDL and higher HDL cholesterol levels, a lower total-to-HDL cholesterol ratio, and lower levels of the pre-clotting protein fibrinogen.[8]

All these findings point to omega-7 as a new chapter in the fight against metabolic and inflammatory disorders that underlie diabetes, cardiovascular disease, obesity, and cancer. Omega-7 is a strong complement to the cardiovascular and lipid benefits of omega-3s.

Proper use of omega-7 could also be a major new anti-aging weapon, since a large element in the aging process is inflammation.

How do I take it? You take it as palmitoleic acid. Numerous studies have shown that a surprisingly tiny dose, less than 250 mg per day over 30 days, produced the significant effects I have described.

The Big Secret Almost Nobody Is Talking About

The world is getting fatter; there is no doubt. But there may be a hidden, very dangerous reason: Environmental toxins.

Studies conducted jointly by researchers at Imperial College London and Harvard University, published in the medical journal *The Lancet*, show that obesity worldwide almost doubled in the decades between 1980 and 2008. [9]

Of course, people are eating too much and exercising too little. Westerners also consume too much of the wrong sort of food, like refined flours and sugars, plus additives including the notorious high fructose corn syrup (HFCS). Far too many empty calories, for sure.

But you may not be aware that there is a virtual epidemic of obesity among six month old infants. Is something else going on? Seems so...

In 2006 scientists at the Harvard School of Public Health reported that the prevalence of obesity in infants under 6 months had risen 73 percent since 1980. "This epidemic of obese 6-month-olds," as endocrinologist Robert Lustig of the University of California, San Francisco, calls it, poses a problem for conventional explanations of the fattening of America.

"Since they're eating only formula or breast milk, and never exactly got a lot of exercise, the obvious explanations for obesity don't work for babies," he points out. "You have to look beyond the obvious."[10]

What is it causing fat babies?

"The evidence now emerging says that being overweight is not just the result of personal choices about what you eat, combined with inactivity," says Retha Newbold of the National Institute of Environmental Health Sciences (NIEHS) in North Carolina, part of the National Institutes of Health (NIH). "Exposure to environmental chemicals during development may be contributing to the obesity epidemic."

As the *Washington Post* reported in 2007: several recent animal studies suggest that environmental exposure to widely used chemicals may also help make people fat. [11]

We've all heard about xenoestrogens in the environment and other hormone or endocrine disruptors, as they are known. Certain chemicals, like bisphenol A and tributyltin, have been shown to trigger fat-cell activity—a process scientists call adipogenesis.

The picture which is emerging is that when humans are exposed to these chemicals, even while in the womb, genetic changes occur which are then irreversible and with the individual for life. It's got the proportions of a tragedy.

But it's worse: it appears there is a growing number of chemicals which seem to have the specific side-effect of causing obesity...

Obesogens

Professor Bruce Blumberg coined the term "obesogens" (which means *makers of obesity*) for this type of chemical which triggers fat cell activity and the name seems to have caught on.

The problem is, potential obesogens are very common in our environment, in our food and in the water supply. One study by the Centers for Disease Control and Prevention (USA) found bisphenol A, in 95 percent of the people tested, at levels at or above those that we know affect developmental growth in animals. In 2003, U.S. industry consumed about 2 billion pounds (1 million net tons) of bisphenol A. It's an ingredient in polycarbonate plastics used in many products, including but not confined to refillable water containers, plastic food wrappings and even baby bottles.

Bisphenol A is approved by the Food and Drug Administration for use in consumer products, and the agency says the amount of bisphenol A or tributyltin that might leach from products is too low to be of concern. This is criminally dangerous and deliberate disinformation by a government body, which is notorious for protecting its industry friends and not the public it is supposed to serve.

As well as criminal, it's stupid. Because here we are talking about a hormone-like action. Hormones only require vanishingly small traces to have their effect (estrogen dominance in women is not a measure of toxic levels but of hormonally-active levels)

Jerry Heindel, a top official of the National Institute of Environmental Health Sciences (NIEHS), described the suspected link between obesity and exposure to hormone disrupters, as "plausible and possible."

I say it goes beyond "possible". There's science: infant mice exposed to obesogens became obese adults and remained obese even on reduced calorie and increased exercise regimes. Retha Newbold, (NIEHS) in North Carolina, carried out research in which newborn mice were given low doses of hormone-mimicking compounds (equivalent to what people are exposed to in the environment). *In six months, the exposed mice were 20 percent heavier and had 36 percent more body fat than unexposed mice.*

This is very strange because normally we would consider body weight to be a function of calories in, minus calories out. Yet the mice were not eating more than normal mice or moving around less; this was monitored especially carefully. Here's proof if it were needed that it's not just about how much you eat, or even what you eat, but that hormones do play a part.

As further proof, in 2005 scientists in Spain reported that the more pesticides children were exposed to as fetuses, the greater their risk of being overweight as toddlers. And last January scientists in

Belgium found that children exposed before birth to higher levels of PCBs and DDE (the breakdown product of the pesticide DDT) were fatter than those exposed to lower levels.

Neither study proves causation, but they "support the findings in experimental animals," says Newbold. They "show a link between exposure to environmental chemicals ... and the development of obesity."

The chemical industry always fights science like this, with every trick in the book, not excluding outright lies, causing deliberate confusion. But only the media are fooled and print what they are told, rather than the facts the public needs to know.

But you need to understand the scale and impact of this problem. If you've ever tried to lose weight and found it difficult, this could be part of the reason why. (another possibility is low thyroid function; the most under-diagnosed health problem out there and a definite cause of overweight).

If you suspect problems associated with xenobiotics, such as unexplained weight gain, breast cancer, prostate problems, loss of libido, depression, mood swings, etc., you must get rid of onboard xenobiotic chemicals, any of which might be obesogens in your body. How?

The best I know is regular repeat far-infrared saunas. You sweat out the xenobiotics (so be careful to shower toxins off your skin, after every session in the sauna).

Reduce ongoing exposure: Go organic. Use natural products that are safer for both you and the environment. Eat a diet high in fiber so that toxins are eliminated rather than absorbed. Most of all, eat lots of vegetables, again, preferably organic.

Avoid plastic containers. Especially, never microwave food with a plastic wrap still in place. A recent study showed that microwaving with plastic wrap left in place caused levels 10 million times greater than the FDA acceptable level of the known carcinogen DEHA. This same study also revealed increases in food levels of xenoestrogens.

Take herbs and other supplements that help protect and detoxify the liver such as alpha lipoic acid, milk thistle, and n-acetyl cysteine (NAC).

The finest liver protective in the market today is a range of products based on the citrus fruit bergamot. The science is extensive and incontrovertible. By the time this book gets to print, it is likely the FDA will have approved the most outstanding of these for fatty liver degeneration: a preparation available to you as Dr. Keith's Own® Bergamot Physician's Strength.

You can read more about it here: https://drkeithsown.com/bergamot/

In Summary

You have to offload those dangerous pounds of fat, otherwise you will shorten your life and ruin the quality of the years that you do have, for sure.

There is one important method, which is deeply founded in an historic basis and fully explained by the best of modern science, which we call *intermittent fasting* (section 15).

See, once upon a time, humans were hunter-gatherers. There were no cafes and restaurants, no 24-hour pizzerias, no Starbucks, no McDonalds! You know what I am saying: we just wandered wild and free and foraged for our foods, like other animals. Some days we would eat well; other days we would be forced to go hungry.

It's only since we became a farming society, which in turn enabled cities and civilizations to grow, that we beat the shadow of hunger, once and for all. Even then, a disastrous crop failure would lead to famine, but we had it more or less stitched up.

So Humankind evolved in the presence of intermittent hunger or even short-range famines. If things became really bad, we would just move on and find new hunting and foraging grounds.

You need to understand that there is a hidden bonus in this historical biological picture. We have evolved the knack of feeding off our body fat! When there is no useful food for energy, we just go into ketogenic mode and start to burn our own body! But not just all tissues, we burn fatty tissue in the main.

In this mode, we break down fats and create ketones which, as it happens, are ideal fuel for the brain and muscles. By mimicking history and deliberately engaging in intermittent fasting (bouts of going hungry), we can create ketones and that means burning up fat very quickly!

See section 14 for more details and advice.

PART 2. THE ISSUES

SECTION 8.
SUGAR IS THE REAL ENEMY

This is a book about the science of weight control. But once in a while, science bumps up against politics; not just the politics of power but misleading the population deliberately, fraud and greed. The story of sugar is just such a story.

For decades orthodox science (paid for and propelled by the sugar industry) has been pushing the incorrect story that eating fatty foods is what lies behind overweight and obesity. We have been pressured to eat more carbs and cut down on fat. "Low-fat" has been the tune, as the food industry sang the song of huge profits banked from selling cheap, fluffy carbs as "healthy".

The truth is that it is sugar and carbs that make us fat.

The infamous "seven countries study" by Ancel Keys, published in 1978 and purportedly showing that fats were dangerous was, quite simply, a fake. The evidence was manipulated strongly in favor of the sugar industry. Unfortunately, and undoubtedly by design, it led to the currently held medical opinion regarding the dangers of cholesterol, fats and food substances containing the same.

Keys was trying to prove a position, not get the true facts. So he ignored Denmark and Norway (countries where the diet is rich in fat, but occurrence of heart disease is low) and also Chile (where diet is low in fat, yet occurrence of heart disease is high).

But even though Keys' fraud and the sugar industry trumpery was exposed early this century, there are still those who cling to the old beliefs. To do so, they too are manipulating or ignoring the evidence which is plain to see: eating 60-70% carbs, as we have been told by government "experts", has led to a massive epidemic of obesity. The official "food pyramid" is dangerous. Eating carbs is simply wrong!

On the other hand, eating a diet high in fats (such as the Atkins diet) always results in weight loss, all other factors being equal. Again, there is no real argument. But experts continue to press the point that fats are dangerous. Therefore the Atkins diet must be dangerous. Where's the evidence? There isn't any. Complaints about the Atkins diet are purely theoretical and politically motivated.

Incidentally, an entrancing book called *Eat Fat and Grow Slim* (1958) was published a quarter of a century before Atkins went to press. It was written by my old mentor Richard Mackarness. The message is the same but the earlier writer deserves 95% of the credit.

History Is Pivotal

Why was the sugar industry so keen to shift blame away from their products? Simple, really. Sugar is deadly. It's a killer. Sugar (meaning the refined white product, extracted from plants like sugar cane and sugar beets), is a relatively novel food ingredient for humans. It has only been in our diet since the 16th century.

Technically, this sugar is called sucrose and it is a mixture of 50% glucose and 50% fructose. Invert sugar is a further corruption of this substance.

In 1537, the first sugar refinery was established in Germany. "Refined", of course, sounds desirable, like "sophisticated". The impact of refined sugar on human health started in 17th century and subsequently became very noticeable among mass population, starting 150 years ago.

Until the mid-nineteenth century, diabetes remained a rare disease. As the father of modern medicine, Sir William Osler reported in 1892: of 35,000 outpatients seen at John Hopkins Hospital in Baltimore, only 10 had been diagnosed with diabetes.

Identification of the pre-diabetic state among obese individuals was not known until the 20th Century.

By the start of the present millennium sugar consumption had risen from negligible two hundred years ago, to the point where the average American consumes 130 lbs. of sugar annually (that's the average, some people consume twice that amount).

Overall, since 1900, the amount of sugar that is consumed by the average person has quadrupled. Every year, the entire world consumes about 165 million tons of sugar. That's about 50 lbs. (23 kg.) per person on average.[1]

Pure, White and Deadly

Basically, refinement of sugar means to concentrate its destructive properties and to remove any nutritional worth. There is little enough good in raw sugar; molasses has some minerals, it's true. But purification removes any trace of useful substances.

Don't be fooled by "natural" sugar either. Brown sugar is mostly white sugar, dyed brown to make it look authentic. The only way to get a sugar that is relatively unrefined is to ask for it by name or country of origin: Guyana, Demerara, Muscovado, etc.

Once tasted, sugar has the power to seduce people, who want to come back to that very special delight, time and time again. In reality, it's no different to drug or alcohol addiction. The energy slump when you don't get your sugar "fix" makes you demand more. Few people have the patience or interest to stop sugar altogether and so to break their addiction to it. They don't see the need.

More's the pity, because—get this: **sugar (refined or not) is one of the deadliest foods ever invented**. It's a killer in every sense and has stolen the health of the entire civilized world, driven onwards by false science and denials, money and corruption, ignorance, stupidity and politics.

False Science To Justify Sugar

Sugar is all-natural, say the shills working for the food industry. Yes, sugars do occur in nature. But so do mercury, rabies and opium! That doesn't make them healthy!

They try to tell us that a calorie is just a calorie; it doesn't matter whether it comes from fats or sugars. Fats have the most calories, therefore fats are the enemy is the story they have been spinning for decades. But that is woefully false. There is a completely different metabolic response to a sugar calorie than to, say, a plant protein calorie or meat fatty calorie. The body is unable to properly process sugar calories, as we shall see in this section. Blood sugar control eventually runs haywire and metabolic syndrome, with all its attendant ills (including) diabesity, is inevitable.

Peter Cleave and John Yudkin, two of the most famous British Researchers in the early 1960's, suggested that sugar caused not just diabetes and heart disease but the entire cluster of chronic diseases we see today. If you haven't read Yudkin's famous book *Pure, White and Deadly*, you should.

The response from the sugar industry was to destroy these claims and ruin professor Yudkin's life and achievement, by spreading lies about him and false science. It is a story of heinous dishonesty and evil. The wildfire of deaths and morbidity has gone on since, the flames fanned by industry shills and corrupt dollars.

I'm not just saying this. Forty years on, the evidence has surfaced and you can read the secret correspondence for yourself, revealing the connivance and chicanery that went into damaging the real science, destroying individuals who had integrity and were giving us the true story. The fake science and its supplanting of the truth was done very subtly and cleverly, backed by weak-minded academics, who supported it, or at least failed to expose the sham for what it was.

I repeat: the science is in. It has been for decades. But there is a multi-billion dollar campaign to distract us from the truth.

Make no mistake: sugar makes us fat, sugar is addictive, sugar inflames, sugar rots your teeth, sugar damages your bowel flora, sugar feeds cancer, sugar kills and sugar has no worthwhile merits. It's being sold purely for the profit it generates, despite of all the wholesome and clean science that shows its deadly properties.

What Really Happens

OK, enough of the invective. What does sugar really do inside our bodies?

Take eating a candy bar. As your blood sugar level soars upwards, you feel that 'sugar high'. In response, the hormone insulin floods your system to cope with it all and reduce the blood sugar levels. But the body doesn't get that good news straight away, so we go into an overshoot, and you experience a resulting 'crash' or hypoglycemia (low blood sugar). This is now an emergency situation for our bodies. Low blood sugar makes us feel faint and can't be tolerated. So the sugar addict needs more cookies or a candy bar, to compensate.

Meantime, the body is trying to put things right and secretes the stress hormone, cortisol, which triggers the liver to release its glycogen store (a form of sugar). That is a normal response. But if the individual has already taken a second candy bar or cookie "hit", the two effects together send the blood glucose soaring AGAIN.

More insulin is poured forth and that plummets blood sugar AGAIN. Back to hypoglycemia. And so it goes on in a vicious cycle, up and down, up and down, that you will readily see will soon exhaust insulin reserves and dull the natural response to it. This person is now well on the way to insulin resistance, obesity and eventually diabetes.

So many people are hooked on sugar in this way and they can't ever imagine getting off the rollercoaster. We can feel the similarity of sugar to drugs in our own bodies, even without the backing of studies, which is why we have long used terms like craving, high, rush and crash in relation to sugar.

The new recommendations from the World Health Organisation (WHO) and the UK's official nutrition advisors are that only 5% of your daily calorie intake should consist of added, or 'free' sugars. This equates to approximately seven sugar cubes (30g). Children should have less, they say, no more than 19g a day for children aged 4 to 6 years old (5 sugar cubes), and no more than 24g (6 sugar cubes) for children aged 7 to 10 years old.

That's nuts. I say, if you are trying to look after your health or lose weight, stay completely away from sugar. None. That 5% allowance is just to keep the sugar manufacturers in the loop. 6 sugar cubes a day for a child? Criminal. I say don't allow anything that contains sugar or needs sugar added. Change your or the child's palate! It will save your life.

This is another good reason to avoid manufactured foods of all kinds. They add sugar and keep it hidden. Did you know there is sugar in most breads; they put it in ham and glazes; it's even added to savory foods, like ready-made soups and sauces.

The natural sugar in some fruit, including apples, has increased as new varieties (including Pink Lady, Fuji and Jazz) are bred to satisfy our foolish desire for greater sweetness.

Lay off the sugar if you want to live – it's definitely dangerous!

It is also worth noting that the US Sugar Association (guess who they represent) has previously asserted that it is fine to have up to 25% sugar in your daily diet! 'Advice' like that is going to kill you.

Insulin Resistance

I have hinted that the body eventually stops responding to endless demands for insulin to cope with the excess sugar. That's a state called insulin resistance. Anyone who is 20 lbs. or more overweight has a degree of insulin resistance. Anyone who is obese or has type-II diabetes definitely has marked insulin resistance.

One way we diagnose this is by measuring your blood insulin levels. It can be measured fasting (rather artificial in my view) or measured during a normal day. Taken along with random blood sugar levels, and a fasting blood sugar reading, we can easily interpret what's going on.

If insulin levels are high and blood sugar, even when fasting, is above 120 mg per ml., you have insulin resistance and probable diabetes. If your fasting insulin level is above 25 mIU/L, that could signify pre-diabetes and beginning insulin resistance.

Insulin resistance means your body is not able to dispose effectively of sugars and carbs (which all end up as sugars anyway). As a result, the glucose is turned to fat and stored. That's the last thing we want. It turns the "fat switch" to the ON position (section 6).

Right away, the reader will be able to see that excess sugar consumption leads eventually to insulin resistance, which leads to a sideways shunt of glucose into fat deposits. The final result is inevitable—metabolic syndrome: obesity, blood pressure, diabetes, and cardio-metabolic damage.

Actually, the onset of insulin resistance is getting shorter and shorter, under the onslaught of unnatural manufactured foods. As a result, young kids are now getting insulin resistance and obesity early. Manufacturers of foods rub their hands and gloat at the insane profits they are making.

During the early part of the 21st century, we have seen an alarming increase in type 2 diabetes in youth, concomitant with the rise of obesity in this age group, and in the United States, type 2 diabetes (the obesity type) now accounts for between 8% and 45% of all of the cases of childhood and adolescent diabetes.[2]

Simple Rule: If your waistline is more than 40 inches (men) or 36 inches (women), you have insulin resistance.

Actual healthy recommendations from the British Medical Journal are: 34 inches (88 cm) or less for women; 38 inches (96 cm) or less for men.[3]

Prediabetes

We now commonly see and use the values we call "pre-diabetes". It isn't just a scam (like pre-hypertension is a scam) in order to sell more insulin or metformin. It's real. Left untreated, high blood sugar and high fasting levels of insulin will sooner or later lead to diabetes; usually sooner.

Prediabetes is a wake-up call that you're on the path to diabetes. But it's not too late to turn things around.

It is characterized by too little or too much insulin, when the body stops responding to it (insulin resistance).

There are three objective measures, to establish the diagnosis of pre-diabetes:

1. Hemoglobin A1C. This blood test shows your average blood sugar level for the past 2 to 3 months. It can be used to diagnose pre-diabetes or diabetes. The results are:

- Normal: 5.6% or less
- Prediabetes: 5.7 to 6.4%
- Diabetes: 6.5% or above

2. Fasting plasma glucose test (not eaten for 8 hours)

- Normal if your blood sugar is less than 100 mg/mL.
- Prediabetes if your blood sugar is 100-125
- Diabetes if your blood sugar is 126 or higher

3. Oral glucose tolerance test. After the previous test, you'll drink a sugary solution. Two hours after that, you'll take another blood test. The results are:

- Normal if your blood sugar is less than 140 after the second test
- Prediabetes if your blood sugar is 140-199 after the second test
- Diabetes if your blood sugar is 200 or higher after the second test

Note that these commonly-used 2-hour glucose tolerance tests may not allow sufficient time for abnormalities to develop. For nearly 40 years I have pointed out the weakness in this shortened test and been calling for a 6-hour GTT.

It goes without saying that if you have the warning signs of prediabetes, you MUST ACT. It's no use waiting for the full-on disease condition before you respond. The approach is much the same as for obesity and diabetes. You are probably heading for the full development we call metabolic syndrome.

It puts you at risk of heart attacks, stroke, liver damage, loss of eyesight, non-healing skin ulcers, amputation of the lower limbs and general infirmity for the rest of your life. It also speeds up aging dramatically. You don't want to go there.

At the very least, give up all sugar NOW (see Quick and Simple Diet #2; p. 98). Better still, grasp the nettle and get onto ketogenic dieting (section 14).

Sugar Blocking Herb

A new study has shown that an extract from the leaves of the white mulberry plant (*Morus indica*) – best known as food for silkworms – provides a range of benefits for those who are overweight.

In one study, the active group received 2400 mg of white Japanese mulberry extract, the control group had only placebo. The sub-group which received the mulberry extract lost about 9 kg in 3 months, equal to approximately 10 percent of the initial weight. Moreover, the plasma insulin and GTT curves were lower than those performed at the time of enrolment.

Previous studies have also shown there is a significant blood sugar lowering effect. Mulberry contains a "sugar blocker" (specifically an alpha-glucosidase inhibitor), along with other compounds that appear to improve blood glucose control as well as blood lipids (cholesterol and triglycerides).

Many of these effects of mulberry leaf extract are due to it positively influencing AMPK activity (see Fat Switch, p. 77). [4]

The daily dosage is generally equivalent to 2,400 - 3,000 mg of dried mulberry leaves. Extracts are generally used.

Camu Camu

OK, this is a fruit, not an herb. No matter. It has some sound science.

An extract of camu camu (*Myrciaria dubia*), also known as cacari, or camocamo, a fruit native to the Amazon basin in South America, prevented obesity in mice fed a diet rich in sugar and fat, said researchers at Université Laval and the Quebec Heart and Lung Institute Research Centre. The discovery, which was recently published in the scientific journal *Gut*, suggests that camu camu phytochemicals could play a leading role in the fight against obesity and metabolic disease.

Camu camu is interesting in that it contains 20 to 30 times more vitamin C than kiwis, up to 60 times more than a fresh orange and 5 times more polyphenols than blackberries.

The obvious beneficial health effects of polyphenol-rich berries have been demonstrated previously, according to André Marette, a professor at Université Laval's Faculty of Medicine and principal investigator for the study.

So they decided to test its potential benefits for metabolic syndrome.

The researchers fed two groups of mice a diet rich in sugar and fat for eight weeks. Half the mice were given camu camu extract each day. At the end of the experiment, weight gain in camu camu-treated mice was 50% lower than that observed in control mice and was similar to the weight gain of mice consuming a low-sugar, low-fat diet.

They also found that camu camu improved glucose tolerance and insulin sensitivity and reduced the concentration of blood endotoxins and metabolic inflammation.

This strongly suggests that camu camu will be a useful player in fighting metabolic syndrome, including obesity.

It seems the effect may be caused by a reshaping of the gut microbiome, including a blooming of A. muciniphila and a significant reduction in Lactobacillus bacteria. Even more interesting: transplantation of intestinal microbiota from the camu camu group to germ-free mice lacking an intestinal microbiota temporarily reproduced similar metabolic effects.

The researchers now want to examine whether camu camu produces the same metabolic effects in humans. It's fairly toxic but the use of a controlled extract of the fruit should not pose a problem since it is already commercialized to combat fatigue and stress and stimulate the immune system.

Camu camu is usually ingested as a powder added to drinks or mixed with foods like oatmeal and yogurt. It can also be sprinkled on other types of cereals or foods.

The berry itself is very tart, so powdered versions are popular as supplements to be mixed into drinks and oatmeal to help quell the sourness.

Available on Amazon.

Quick and Simple Diet #2. Give Up All Sugar!

After reading the previous section you should be in no doubt that sugar is the number one enemy. Sugar is totally unnatural, concentrated mischief. It is the number one cause of overweight and obesity. Just give it up. Please!

Believe it or not, you won't miss it after as little as two weeks. Once you break the sugar addiction, even a carrot will start to taste sweet! There's sugar in a wide variety of foods. You just need to get used to the lack of that very intense artificial flavor we call "sweetness".

Which brings me to a very important point: do NOT switch to artificial sweeteners (stevia, sucralose, etc.) These can be a thousand times sweeter than sugar itself. That cannot help you. You want to get rid of the sweetness flavor in your life, not keep your taste buds craving it.

As I said, it will only take a matter of days to break the addiction to that flavor. In two weeks or less you will be revolted by the sweetness levels you once craved!

You will also find your energy levels genuinely rise. The myth that sugar gives us energy is just that: a stupid, ignorant myth. As you have read, taking sugar and initiating a "rush" will momentarily cause a lift in blood sugar. But it won't sustain. The body reacts to this sudden rise and brings it down by secreting insulin. Usually blood levels will plunge below datum and so you feel tired, weak and hungry. We call this condition *hypoglycemia*.

It results in you wanting more sugar; you eat an ice cream, a candy bar or drink a soda. The cycle repeats and you are never satisfied. The inevitable outcome is that your blood sugar control mechanism becomes exhausted, insulin resistance sets in and you feel weak and lethargic all the time.

By this stage, sugary foods and drinks will barely give you a boost. You have wrecked your health and—since insulin is the main hormone which stops blood sugars turning to fat—you pile on the weight. I'm sure I don't need to explain to you that feeling sluggish and slowing down rapidly makes the weight gain problem worse.

This has given rise to a myth: we are overweight because we don't exercise enough.

The Truth: *we don't exercise because we are overweight!*

Sugar has NO redeeming qualities. The wickedly seductive taste gives no hint of the terrible damage that sugar can cause. Give it up! You may find that's all you need to do to lose weight steadily.

For the sake of clarity, let it be said, NO SUGAR means:

- No sugar (no candies, sodas, cookies, muffins, etc)
- No cane juice, no "evaporated" cane juice
- No lactose
- No maltose
- No molasses
- No syrups
- No fructose, especially no HFCS
- No substitute sweeteners
- No honey
- No maple syrup
- No fruit juices (eating fruits in moderation is OK)

Beware also of the trick manufacturers may play, especially here in the USA, of adding sugar to inappropriate products, to make them taste "sweet", so customers keep coming back for more (and so more profits). I'm talking about foods like ham, sausages, bread, baked beans, yoghurt, granola, "energy bars", sauces and condiments (tomato ketchup has over 20 teaspoons of sugar per standard bottle).

Even when a product claims to have "25% less sugar", it doesn't mean it isn't still loaded with a shocking amount; it just translates to rather less.

You need to understand that food manufacturers are trying to trick you. They are not honest and will not help you make healthy choices (review section 3).

PART 2. THE ISSUES

SECTION 9.
COULD THERE BE A HUNGER GENE?

"It's All In My Genes, Doc!"

Years ago, you may remember, obese people would sometimes claim, "It's all in my genes." And everyone would snicker. Perhaps you replied, "Yeah, right!"

We knew it was just an excuse for lack of willpower.

Actually it turns out, many of these people were correct. Hunger, satiety (the feeling of not wanting to eat any more) and obesity are regulated by a growing number of genes. These could make things extremely difficult for the slimmer who is ignorant of their function.

Sounds a silly idea, doesn't it? But in fact scientists first identified the fat mass and obesity associated (FTO) gene in 2007. It was soon nicknamed the "fatso gene". It can lead the body to store fat rather than burn it. The FTO gene is found in 44 per cent of Caucasians but only five per cent of blacks, meaning other genes are clearly at work too (food and exercise still play an important part).

What this really means is not that the individual has a single bad gene, but rather that the he or she has inherited a bad combination from mother and father.

OK, heads down, and let's just take a closer look at this: gene babble is coming at us from all sides, it's important to understand it, at least in principle. Grab a coffee and read the next few paragraphs slowly...

When we say someone has the blue-eyed gene, or the BRCA1 or BRCA2 breast cancer genes, the language is not quite correct and this causes confusion. Genes always come in pairs (with a very few exceptions that need not concern us here).

For every gene, there is a good and bad variant. These two alternatives are called *alleles* (ah-leelahs: the only technical word needed, promise). Let's play around with this: say our gene has a good variant G and an unhealthy variant U. We could have got a G from both parents: the combination would be GG. That's good news. Or we could have got a U from both parents: UU. That's pretty unhealthy. Then I'm sure you've already jumped ahead and figured out we could have one of each: GU. With that combination you might have problems, or maybe not.

So you will appreciate that to say someone "Has the BRCA1 gene" is really sloppy talk. It is more correct to say that the person has got the two bad alleles for BRCA1. You will hear even scientists using language like "two copies of the FTO gene', when they mean two bad alleles for the FTO gene.

This is a crucial concept. If you sign up for a gene profile with companies like *23andME, Fitgenes* or *SmartDNA* you will receive a report which is typically coded red-green-amber. Red means you have both bad alleles, amber means you have one of each and green means you have the two good alleles.

If you have the red combination of any gene, you need to deal with it to protect your health. Even if you have the amber combination, it's still a good idea to work to switch off that gene.

Altering genes in this way—tuning out the bad ones and strengthening the good ones—we call epigenetics. More of that later in this section.

OK, let's dive in!

The FTO Gene

So far, inheriting two copies of the FTO is the most common genetic contributor to overweight and obesity in the world today. It is estimated to affect 1 billion people worldwide. But how big a deal is it?

With two bad alleles of this gene (red pairing), you are much more likely to feel hunger, even after eating, says researcher Rachel Batterham, MD, PhD, of the University College London and head of Obesity and Bariatric Services at the UCL Hospital. Apparently, that affects one in six people. One of the bad consequences of the red pairing is high levels of the hormone ghrelin, which increases hunger, even after eating (see section 4).

From previous studies, it is known that around 40% to 70% of a person's BMI is inherited. That's not as bad as it sounds; things are more complex than just percentages. Overall, the role of any single gene in obesity is not major. However, if all the obesity-related genes are considered together, the effect would probably be very significant.

Unfortunately, the FTO turns out to be more crucial than your average gene. Since 2007, it has been known that people who carry two bad copies of the FTO gene are 70% more likely to be overweight or obese. These people will eat more calories and prefer high-calorie foods, according to research. They are not just over eaters but also respond more sluggishly to satiety cues. They are thus the classic binge eaters.

Even healthy-weight people with two copies of the FTO gene were found to respond to high-calorie food images more than those with the low-risk variant (whether they had eaten or not). Brain scans confirmed this important finding, showing increased activity in regions of the brain known to regulate appetite, reward, and motivate behavior.

It is important to note that people with the FTO double whammy are also more prone to inflammation. One of the principle markers for inflammation, C-reactive protein (CRP), is 14% higher in men, 12% higher in women per FTO allele (Fisher 2009). You will remember that inflammation is a major problem in obesity, first for the damage it does and secondly because it blocks weight loss (section 7).

What is obvious is that lifestyle modifications, such as diet control, exercise and even behavioral therapy will be helpful, indeed probably necessary, for people who have the double FTO. These individuals have a tougher path to weight loss.

MC4R

Melanocortin 4 receptor (MC4R). This is a beast of a gene (red variant). It's the one gene that can be harmful all by itself, never mind interacting with other obesity genes.

It creates havoc with eating habits. The MC4 receptor is a key signaling center for control of food intake, especially in women. It leads them to consume more food and more fat. It is second only to the FTO for the trouble it causes but the two together make a deadly combination.

Unfortunately, it lowers the person's response to leptin, the appetite hormone that is supposed to signal "enough" and kill the desire for food (see section 4).

MC4R's action is mainly via the hypothalamus, where energy homeostasis, food intake and body weight are mostly regulated, especially in women.

Make sure you get this in the test panel if you go for genetic testing. It's routine at most labs and you wouldn't want to be left guessing, if you have weight issues.

This is very important to people of Indian and Asian ancestry; it is associated with extreme states of hyperinsulinemia (very high insulin levels, a marker for diabetes and insulin resistance). It leads to increased waist circumference, high fat mass and obesity.

Finally, MC4R is the number one culprit for childhood obesity. If your child is seriously pudgy or diagnosed obese, get it checked.

ADRβ2 and ADRβ3 (ADR beta 2 and 3)

These two are probably the next two most important fat genes, after FTO and MC4R, since they regulate lipid (fat) metabolism via the adrenal hormones adrenalin and noradrenalin (epinephrine and norepinephrine).

ADRβ2 is a receptor found mainly in the nervous system, brain, kidney and muscle. The beneficial double (green pairing) turns on this receptor. In doing so this activates the mechanisms of energy regulation through heat generation (thermogenesis) and breakdown of fats for muscle energy work to prevent obesity.

It is an interesting aside all the Kenyan marathon runners, who have dominated this event in the Olympics, have the green pairing and are famously lean, as well as fit.

In contrast, the orange or red pairings are associated with marked obesity (Martinez, 2003; Arner, 1999) and also larger fat cells. All fats in our body are stored in cells called adipocytes. We'd like them as tiny as possible, obviously, so they can hold very little fat; so BIG is bad news. The orange or red variants are also markedly associated with belly fat in men, especially men with low HDL cholesterol levels.

But for women it's bad news too. With the orange, and especially the red pairing, women have a significantly higher carbohydrate intake (49% of total energy intake). So if gene testing shows you have the red combination, it will be the low carb diets for you!

ADRβ3 is also involved in regulating energy metabolism, via thermogenesis. The red pairing puts you at risk of insulin resistance and metabolic syndrome (diabesity). It's a bigger problem for women in that it is associated with estrogen levels. So if you want to fight this one, make sure you get your hormones tested too. Estrogen dominance, as it is called, will push you quickly into overweight and eventually obesity.

One other thing you need to know: with the bad coupling for ADRβ3, diet and exercise don't result in good loss of body fat. Bummer!

UCP1 and UCP3

UCP is short for uncoupling proteins, which are a special class of proteins in the mitochondria. They have been found to play a major role in energy balance and have become important in the field of thermogenesis (heat production), obesity, diabetes and free-radical biology. These are now considered candidate genes for obesity and insulin resistance—in other words, diabesity.

UCP1 is prevalent in brown adipose tissue, which you may heard of. It is associated with the ability to burn energy and stay lean.

UCP1 is highly regulated by the sympathetic nervous system and activation of ADRβ3 increases it.

UCP3 on the other hand is involved in the regulation of fats as fuel and not just via thermogenesis. UCP3 is expressed most abundantly in skeletal and heart muscle. It also stimulated good brown adipose tissue to release energy as heat. This is an important defence against obesity (Liu, 2005).

Generally the red and orange variants mean lower energy states and a tendency to store energy as fat. Quick tip: the 2-5 diet works well for you (two 500 calories days per week: see section 15).

Fat Absorption Gene FAB2

It's good to know that fat absorption is also regulated by a gene: FAB2. Double green is good. Red and orange are associated with increased fat absorption and therefore an increased risk of being overweight. It also means a rise in fatty acid oxidation. That's bad news too because it impairs the action of insulin. In section 8 you will have read that low insulin or insulin resistance (either) will block cellular uptake of glucose and it is then switched to fat instead.

Either way, these are pre-diabetic changes. BMI is up and body fat, especially abdominal fat, is also up.

One good way to start losing weight is to turn off the bad pairing. That means you'll absorb less fat from your intestine.

The poor versions of FAB2 are associated with increased inflammation, once again blocking the ability to lose weight by making simple changes. Individuals carrying the red pairing will find themselves very resistant to weight loss.

You will have to deal with this. You are also an individual who benefits from a low-fat diet. I suggest you keep your calorie intake to around 1,500 kcal per day.

PPARγ (PPAR gamma)

While we are on the subject of fat storage, let's consider another gene, the PPARγ. This little puppy controls genes associated with the uptake of lipids by fat cells (adipocytes). It also controls the number and size of fat cells. As I said, small is beautiful; it means the cells will hold less fat.

Unfortunately, the red and orange variants mean an increased risk of obesity, diabetes and inflammation (PPARγ is recognized as a central inhibitor of intestinal inflammation). Also the unlucky individuals have a higher food efficiency; that's not as good as it sounds. It means they need less intake to maintain a stable weight.

If you are a female, you'll gain weight more quickly and—worst of all—you will rebound faster and further when you start to pile it back on.

Eating anything becomes a weight gain nightmare!

Exercizing is good for this one, it lowers insulin resistance. Also zinc is critical to PPARγ gene expression (Meerani, 2003). Remember, this is a gene we want to do it's job, not keep it suppressed.

We'll discuss interventions in a moment. But first...

Vitamin D

This may surprise you. But in fact vitamin D is a monster vitamin that beneficially affects at least nine hundred genes. These nine hundred genes then exert their effects on target tissues such as bone, skeletal muscle, immune system, skin, nervous tissue and endothelial tissues (lining of the arteries).

Vitamin D also has a powerful effect in quenching inflammation. Two important inflammation markers, so-called C reactive protein (CRP) and TNFα, are quickly raised when vitamin D levels are low. I have repeatedly referred to this important issue; inflammation running in your body will virtually block weight loss. It's that important.

Yet almost half the world's population are deficient. In fact vitamin D deficiency is a major global health problem.

Vitamin D is critical to

- Alzheimer's and dementia
- Autism spectrum disorder (ASD)
- Autoimmune disorders
- Bone density
- Cancer
- Cardiovascular disease
- Heavy metal toxicity (lead, mercury, etc.)
- Insulin resistance/diabetes/metabolic syndrome
- Inflammatory bowel disease
- Mental health
- Obesity
- Psoriasis

You will quickly see then that vitamin D levels are crucial to slimmers. Lack of vitamin D leads to obesity. But then it becomes a double whammy because what little vitamin D is in your system gets locked up in the fatty tissue, compounding the problem.

Vitamin D receptors are equally important and their function is controlled by two more genes: VDR and VDR2. Before I discuss these two, let me offer some quick tips:

- 80-90% of your vitamin D intake will come from sunlight.
- 10-20% from dietary intake (ordinary dietary sources usually provide about 100 IU daily).[1]

Rich dietary sources are oily fish, such as salmon, mackerel, herring and sardines. You should play safe and supplement with a minimum of 2,000 IU daily. I take 4,000 IU daily.

If your doctor will play along with you, get a blood test and we aim for serum levels of 25-hydroxyvitamin D or 25(OH)D of around 50 – 70 ng/ml. You might even want to push it on to 80-100 ng/ml. Below 50 ng/ml is considered deficiency. I have seen levels as low as 30 ng/ml in individuals who simply don't eat well. That's dangerous (cancer and cardiovascular problems).

Note that a serious infection or any other rampant inflammation process, like autoimmune disease, will plummet your vitamin D levels.

VDR and VDR2

These receptors control many factors, including:

- Inflammation
- Immune function
- Oxidative stress
- Bone density
- Body weight
- Insulin secretion response to sugar and glucose

Therefore you definitely want the green combo. If you are not so lucky, I'll tell you what to do shortly.

The red combo is associated with an average of 20 lbs. weight excess (9 kilos) and about 4 extra units on BMI.

Not only weight gain but other risk factors come into play, such as coronary artery disease, bad blood fats, blood pressure and calcification. Forget what you've read about calcium supplements: calcium is a deadly sign of aging—crumbling joints, hardening of the arteries, aging of the brain, and a host of other stiffness factors. What you want is magnesium; we want less calcium.[2]

AMY1 "The Atkins Gene"

Recently isolated, the AMY1 is probably the number one obesity gene. You need to understand why it is a potential problem and you need to get your "AMY1 copy number". What does that mean? We all have copies of certain genes, sometimes many copies. The AMY1 gene, which expresses as amylase, an enzyme for digesting starch, is one such multiple gene.

Basically the science is saying this: The more copies of the AMY1 gene you have, the less likely you are to be obese. Individuals with fewer than 4 copies are 8 times more likely to be obese than those with 9 or more copies.

AMY1 copy number had a stronger association with BMI than variants of the "Fatso" (FTO). Some wit suggested we call it the "Atkins gene", since avoiding starch is what Atkins was telling us for decades.

A low AMY1 copy number is typical of the hunter-gatherer eater. He or she should be following the Atkins high-fat, low-carb approach (HFLC). Starch and sugars are a no-no; these are farmer foods, not hunter-gatherer foods.

You need to know your AMY1 copy number. Remember, it never changes through your life. Only the "expression" of a gene can be changed.

But this test can tell us more. If you are significantly overweight and your AMY1 copy number is good (9 or more) then one thing is certain: inflammation is what is driving the weight problem, not what you eat.

See, a person with a high copy number should be able to eat plenty of starch, without gaining weight. If food goes straight to your hips and elsewhere, you know for sure you have rampant inflammation running in your body (section 7) and you need to get it down.

Omega-3s (highly anti-inflammatory) will help you lose weight faster and more surely than by taking weight loss pills or counting calories. Other natural anti-inflammatory substances include curcumin (from Turmeric), ginger, alpha lipoic acid and Cat's Claw. Taking an enzyme mix which includes Bromelain and Papain is beneficial too.

Finally, don't forget to test yourself for inflammatory foods, using the guide in section 5. Food allergies and intolerance are probably the number one cause of systemic inflammation. That's because we put so much food into our bodies.

Genomic Testing

If you have had the least difficulty losing weight or keeping it off, I highly recommend you get genomic testing. All that I have written in this section will then become meaningful to you. You don't need your whole genome sequencing and, in any case, the cost would be prohibitive. Just 50 – 60 key genes will be very revealing, of which the dozen or so I have pinpointed above would be very helpful to you. At the time of writing, the cost for such testing has come down to under $500.

The test is easy to administer. You empty your mouth and wait for 30 minutes. Then swab the inside of your cheek for at least one minute, break off the stick and drop the swab end into a tube, which is sealed and shipped in the post. It's a very durable sample and will last many weeks, so there is no rush as with, for example, a blood samples—and none of the biological specimen regulation hassles.

Don't be swayed by how many genes the lab claims to test. The bigger issue is quality, not quantity; meaning you want results that are totally trustworthy. More of that in a moment.

There are a number of test labs which deal directly with the public. This will change over the life of this book. When you are ready, do your due diligence and decide on the best option available in your territory. If you engage a health practitioner there will be more choice. Unfortunately, the world lab I trust the most will only work via practitioners trained and certified by them.

They are Australian-based (Melbourne) but that is no limitation these days, when you can get a skype consultation anywhere in the world. The company is called FitGenes (www.FitGenes.com). Their rivals SmartDNA (www.SmartDNA.com) are also in Australia. These two companies are the best so far for accuracy. You don't get as much practical advice from SmartDNA (or rather someone will just read the report to you) but that's no problem for readers of this book.

By the end of this section you will be HOT on interpreting and fixing obesity genes!

Check out below.

Other labs: USA 23and ME (23andME.com). After you get your results you want to go to Genetic Genie LLC (wwwgeneticgenie.com) where you can upload your data and this website service will tell you your methylation status.

Methylation is an important physiological process, by which we turn good and bad genes on and off. It means to donate methyl groups, one carbon and three hydrogen (-CH3). You can do this with vitamins B1, B6 and B12, and folic acid. Other suppliers of the methyl group include TMG (trimethylglycine) and S-adenosyl methionine (SAMe)

Turning Off Bad Genes

It's important to understand that the results of genetic tests are not always "yes or no" for the presence or the risk of developing a condition, which make interpretations and explanations difficult. In most cases, symptoms occur as a result of interaction among multiple genes and the environment — for example, a person's lifestyle, the foods they eat, and the substances to which they're exposed, like sunlight, chemicals, and tobacco. The interplay of these factors in contributing to health and disease can be very complex.

Nevertheless, I have already hinted that we can "tune out" or tune down bad genes. If you have been tested and find you have the FTO, MC4R genes or any of the others that influence weight control, you will need to learn this skill.

Surprising as it may seem, it is not all that difficult. You will have a different emphasis for changing your diet than just counting calories or carbs! You will be working on a gene control strategy.

Two things I can say right away: a good diet, avoiding allergy foods (inflammatory foods) is probably your number one salvation. All kinds of bad stuff turns off and "good genes" light up. See section 5 for comprehensive advice on getting this right.

Secondly, methylation is crucial for epigenetics. Methylation (above) can silence or tone down genes.

Meantime, let me set up interventions for each of the major obesity/fat genes described above.

FTO

The Mediterranean Diet is unquestionably the best diet for you to hold your weight down.[3]

Even so you will have to downsize portions and lower calories. Any slip up and you could trigger binge eating. You need to be careful and keep yourself on a rope.

I have already indicated that people with FTO risk variants are more likely to overeat due to low satiety. This includes:

- eating larger portions (more calories)
- preferring calorie-dense foods that are high in fat and sugar, such as biscuits, cakes, pastries, cheese, fatty meats, etc.
- enjoying palatable foods (mostly appetizers, desserts and snacks) after already having eaten a meal; and
- snacking more frequently.

You must work hard to stamp out these traits in yourself.

Guard against addictions and bingeing by following the advice about food allergy, section 5. Food addictions you cannot afford!

Exercise is crucial. 60 minutes/day of moderate to vigorous physical activity will cancel out the effects of the FTO gene.[4] It's important to you. There is a direct association between leisure-time activity and lowered death rate from heart attack.

MC4R

You guys too have satiety problems. This gene will drive you relentlessly, making you want to over eat. About 49-56% of people have mild low satiety and 13-15% have severe low satiety. The percentage of those with severe low satiety is higher in overweight and obese (49-55%) populations. Once your weight goes up, it is hard to get it down.

All I wrote for the FTO gene applies to you too.

But you can help satiety by eating more fatty foods. Fat is satisfying and gives that full feeling. This helps tone down the MC4R. But researchers are worried that long-term high fat eating (as with Atkins) will lower methylation of the gene. That means MC4R will again re-assert itself; hunger and munching on the rise and that problem of rebounding back to heavier than before you started. Recognize your pattern?

You need to master methylation supplements and use them to counter the effects of high-fat dieting, which remains your best option.

ADRβ2 and ADRβ3

Both these genes mean the body will respond far better to exercise than to food restriction for weight loss. In fact with the red or orange variants of ADRβ2, dieting does not have any real impact on fat mass, waist circumference or resting metabolic rate but did result in the loss of lean muscle. That's a bummer. [5]

Choose a low carb approach, instead of a low calorie approach. Otherwise carbs will drive up your insulin levels. That's bad.

Carriers of ADRβ3 red variant lost more fat, and twice as much belly fat, in response to exercise as did the green variant for this gene.

What this is saying is you need to move more. If you are sedentary in work habits, you need to compensate for that. Join a gym, take up tennis, get a bicycle or do something. Sitting still is a disaster for you!

You also need to get checked regularly for your glucose and insulin stats. Diabetes is always just around the corner—though you don't have to go there!

UCP1 and UCP3

With UCP1 red variant it is important to get your thyroid checked. You may be at special risk of thyroid slowing. Low-dose progesterone should help (see section 11) but avoid synthetic progestogens at all costs.

Seaweed is good. Drink green and white tea with epicatechins. [6]

Also you need to top up well on vitamin Am the retinoic (hormonal) form. It's known to up-regulate UCP1.

UCP3, fasting and slam dieting works well for you, due to changes in blood fatty acids; no negatives.

Sugars and carbs are bad for you because that lowers fat metabolism which, as I have just said, does help. So no sodas or jet drinks at the gym and especially no drinks sweetened with corn syrup.

Exercizing up-regulates UCP3 expression, not directly but via changes in blood fatty acids (meaning, if the blood fatty acids don't in fact change, there is no up-regulation of UCP3).

FAB2

Aerobic exercise, 3 times a week is required.

At the same time you need to lower your fat intake. Interestingly, your FAB2 expression goes down as you avoid fats and rises if you bring fats into your diet. It's on an as-needed basis.

Keep your calories, as I said, to around 1500- 1600 max.

This is a bad gene for diabetes. Be sure to get checked up annually by your doctor. It can also increase your serum triglycerides, one of the "bad fats" that cardiologists worry about.

You'll want to know about leptin levels, since they operate against you with this gene (section 4).

PPARγ

You will want to exercise regularly. Expression of PPARγ doubled after patients completed a 12-week exercise program.

Despite the presence of the red or orange variants, subjects were able to dramatically improve their insulin resistance levels after exercise. That in turn makes it less likely you will develop metabolic syndrome. That's great news. You still need to get your weight down, of course.

You can help yourself with targeted nutrition:

Zinc is a critical part of PPARγ gene expression. You need to supplement this. Take 50 mg of the gluconate or oratate form (if you want to follow only the elemental zinc, take about 15 mg).

Conjugated linoleic acid (CLA) can induce PPARγ expression but it is dependent on the presence of sufficient zinc. Studies have shown that CLA reduces body fat while preserving muscle tissue, and may also increase your metabolic rate. A study published in the American Journal of Clinical Nutrition found that individuals who took 3.2 grams of CLA per day had a drop in fat mass of about 0.2 pounds each week (that's about one pound a month) compared to those given a placebo. OK, not a massive effect but healthful, nonetheless.

Since CLA cannot be manufactured in the human body, you must get it from your diet by consuming high-quality dietary sources such as grass-fed beef.

Finally, sulforaphane increases the beneficial effect of PPARγ. See the recommendations for VDR and VDR2 (next) for very important instructions of getting the right kind of sulforaphane. 99% of what's out there for sale is junk and will not, cannot, work for you.

VDR and VDR

The three important strategies are:

1. to UP your supplementation of vitamin D to mega-doses; as I said, at least 2,000 IU daily. Better is 4,000 – 5,000 IU.
2. Get some progesterone (yes, even guys)
3. And take sulforaphane.

Supplementation

Medscape reports that the present data indicate that in obese and overweight people with vitamin D deficiency, vitamin D supplementation aids weight loss and enhances the beneficial effects of a reduced-calorie diet. The researchers suggest that all overweight and obese people should have their vitamin D levels tested.

Progesterone For Weight Loss

This is not a crazy idea: estrogen is associated with weight gain; progesterone mitigates the negative effects of excess estrogen (estrogen dominance).

Science is now showing that progesterone can upregulate the VDR genes. This is mostly studied in relation to bone density but is exactly the kind of result we want. [7]

You can learn more about using progesterone to tone down estrogen dominance in section 11.

Sulforaphane Know-How

Sulforaphane up-regulates vitamin D receptors. Now here's the catch: suppliers everywhere will sell you brocolli seed extract or sulforaphane glucosinolate and claim it's the same as sulforaphane. It's not! Neither of these will liberate any useful levels of sulforaphane. [8]

You need preparations which state clearly and unequivocally on the label that BOTH glucoraphanin is present AND the enzyme myrosinase which activates it. In effect that means whole food Brussels sprouts powder.

Warning: I went to Amazon and the first 18 returns for "glucoraphanin" were worthless. Use the search word "myrosinase". Even then, the only two valuable products I found were Vitalica Plus, Enzyme Activated Broccoli Supplement and Myrosinase activated SGS BroccoMax by Jarrow Formulas.[9]

Summing It Up

OK, now do you see why we need some science in this field? People peddling fixed diet plans are kidding the world. Most of them don't care anyway and never respond to commentary that their plan might not work for many people. Their aim is to hype and hustle and make as much money as possible, before their particular bubble bursts.

Genomic testing is certainly not the only way forward for those who are having difficulty finding the right eating pattern. But it will help you eliminate some of the confusion about what you should eat and what part exercise plays.

Taken in conjunction with all the other scientifically demonstrated barriers to slimming explained in this book, you will find yourself in a far more powerful position to fight the flab!

Quick and Simple Diet #3. Avoid All "White Foods"

After the "Cut Up Foods" Quick and Simple Diet #1, and the "Give Up Sugar" diet #2, here's another quickie you can institute right away, without looking up any information!

Just avoid white foods. Not just refined white sugar: all of them! These foods are almost entirely unnatural or processed, so it's a way to hit back at manufacturers. Many celebrities including Cameron Diaz and Oprah have endorsed this simple diet.

White foods are as follows: breads, refined flours of all grains (especially wheat and corn), all cornstarch derivatives, rice, white sugar, high fructose corn syrup (which they now try to re-label corn sugar), milk, potatoes, pasta, pastry and pizza dough.

Tortillas, tamales, nachos and empenadas are not necessarily white but come under the same bad foods category, because of the wheat flour and/or cornstarch rule.

However naturally white foods, such as onions, cauliflower, turnips and white beans are allowed because they are not refined.

The difference between refined white foods and their healthier counterparts is processing and fiber. Most white carbs start with flour from grain that has been refined by stripping off the outer layer, where the fiber is located. These nutrient-stripped foods do not satisfy the appetite well and can lead to excess snacking.

Vitamins and/or minerals are frequently added back to enrich the refined product but the amounts added are pathetic, compared to what is destroyed by processing. Pay no attention to the "vitamin-enriched" claim (page 40).

Including milk, might surprise you but milk is an unnatural food for humans. More importantly, it has a high sugar content (lactose) and will definitely disturb your blood glucose balance.

Note that skimmed milk is worse, not better. There is less fat but proportionately more sugar. More than that: milk seems to trigger a disproportionate release of insulin, considering its relatively low carbohydrate content and people at risk of insulin resistance should probably limit their milk consumption until more studies are conducted on the subject, according to the authors of a 2005 study in "British Journal of Nutrition". [10]

PART 2. THE ISSUES

SECTION 10. PILLS AND HERBS

The idea of swallowing a magic potion and the pounds will melt away is a dream that excites countless slimmers. But is there such a thing? Can we ever stop worrying about what we eat and just enjoy limitless food, while some miracle seed or plant does all the clean-up work for us? No.

It's never going to happen. Given that the problem with overweight is that the person has an unhealthy lifestyle and diet, matters are never going to come to rights until he or she develops better habits. That's a must. You know it's true.

But that doesn't stop us seeking out aids that make the process of losing weight quicker or easier! The question is: can popping pills or powders work? Yes and No. Some touted slimming aids do have good science, others are little better than a scam, some criminally so. Lets start with herbs...

A number of herbs do seem to stand up to trustworthy scientific appraisal and they may help. I'm thinking, for example, of *Undaria pinnatifida*, a kelp, also known as wakame.

Wakame (*Undaria pinnafitida*)

This plant extract contains significant levels of a compound called fucoxanthin, a remarkable protein, proven to increase metabolic rate and cause cells to burn fat for energy—not just during exercise, but at rest. So more reason than ever to include the regular exercise!

In a test group, people taking fucoxanthin combined with pomegranate seed oil lost an average of 15 pounds in four months, compared to just 3 pounds in the control group. [1]

African mango (*Irvingia gabonensis*)

Another well-studied and proven supplement is a West African herb called *Irvingia gabonensis*. After 10 weeks, test subjects taking this extract dropped an average of 28 pounds and shed 6 inches around their waist.

The results were published in a respectable online journal *Lipids in Health and Disease*. [2]

FOX News picked up the story from Reuters when the study hit the media. [3]

Garcinia cambogia (hydroxycitric acid or HCA)

Several studies have shown that *Garcinia cambogia* can play an important role in the regulation of fat metabolism. It can help prevent the liver from turning the sugar and carbohydrates in food into fat. This effect is specially attributed to hydroxycitric acid (HCA).

In addition, *G. cambogia* has been found to stimulate the production of serotonin, which encourages a feel-good factor, inhibits the production of the 'stress hormone' cortisol and can prevent the person concerned from wanting to over-eat.

Several studies have found that the administration of G. cambogia extract is associated with body weight and fat loss in both experimental animals and humans. According to a study from Georgetown University Medical Center, people who took the *Garcinia Cambogia* supplement for 8 weeks lost an average of 16.5 pounds without additional diet or exercise.

Another study published in *Nutrition Research* found that people taking G. cambogia extract lost an average of 6.7 percent of their total body weight (12.3 percent of their total body fat) with no side effects whatsoever. However, other studies have failed to find this effect, so caution is advised.

Unfortunately, even the positive studies were conducted on small samples and mainly in the short term. None of them have shown whether these effects persist beyond 12 weeks of intervention. Therefore, there is still little evidence to support the potential long-term benefits of *G. cambogia* and other herbal extracts.

With regard to toxicity and safety, it is important to note that except in rare cases, studies conducted in experimental animals have not reported increased mortality or significant toxicity. Furthermore, at the doses usually administered, no differences have been reported in terms of side effects or adverse events in humans, between individuals treated with G. cambogia and controls.

Garcinia Cambogia and Green Coffee Bean Extract Combination

There is a further interesting twist to the G. cambogia story. In the US it has formed part of a hot craze amongst people trying to lose weight, since it appears to be even more effective when combined with Green Coffee Bean Extract.

One study that has been published in the journal entitled *Diabetes, Metabolic Syndrome and Obesity* found that people taking Green Coffee Bean extract lost an average of 8.4% of their total body weight and 4.4% of their total body fat, all without making any changes to their diet.

Add that kind of efficacy to the potential effects of G. cambogia and it may not be surprising that recent reports on the use of hydroxycitric acid and Green Coffee Chlorogenic Acid Extract suggests that the combination of the two may be far more effective. Worth exploring further by those who are interested in using natural supplements to boost weight loss.

But... please... stick to advice everywhere else in the book, about eating better and adopting a healthier, less sedentary lifestyle!

Eat Curries! (Turmeric)

Traditionally, no-one would have thought that curry was slimming. If there is any doubt, consider the Indian nation, which has one of the highest obesity and diabetes rates outside the USA.

But there is a lie in this slick observation: turmeric (curry ingredient), helps you lose weight! Curries are good for the slimmer. It's probable that it blocks "hunger signals" between your stomach and brain. So the overweight probably comes from the grains (chapatti and rice)... or the beer!

Turmeric (*Curcuma longa*) is the plant which gives rise to the spice curcumin. This substance, and others like it (called curcuminoids), have a whole range of health benefits, from improving your skin and preventing wrinkles, to boosting the immune system, protecting liver health and lots of science shows it protects against cancer.

It is definitely effective against obesity and has enjoyed a traditional reputation in this regard for centuries. But why is this? Researchers at the Jean Mayer USDA Human Nutrition Research Center on Aging at Tufts University discovered that curcumin, actually prevents the growth of fat cells in mice.[4]

So I don't think it's unreasonable to put turmeric in your diet a couple of times a week. Learn to make tasty Indian style dishes but hold on the nan breads and rice! Instead, make a "rice substitute" by slightly over-boiling cauliflower and then mashing it, just like you would potato. It comes out with surprisingly fluffy "grains" that easily fool the palate, once the curry portion is dropped over it! (the cauli needs a little over-cooking because you cannot mash al-dente cauliflower).

This pretend rice has no carbs and very few calories indeed.

Here are some other ways in which turmeric can boost your health, making it a terrific all-round cookery flavor.

It boosts the immune system, which can have enormous impact, including even reducing your risk of cancer (curcumin has emerged as a potent multimodal cancer-preventing agent, with literally hundreds of published studies appearing in the global scientific literature [5]

Turmeric seems to help prevent Alzheimer's disease. Among Indian people aged 70 to 79, the rate is less than one-quarter that of the United States.

To sum up the benefits of turmeric and curcumin, an overview published in *Advanced Experimental Medical Biology* in 2007 stated that, "Curcumin has been shown to exhibit antioxidant, anti-inflammatory, antiviral, antibacterial, antifungal, and anticancer activities and thus has a potential against various malignant diseases, diabetes, allergies, arthritis, Alzheimer's disease and other chronic illnesses." [6]

Add all that to the weight control potential of turmeric and you will see why I recommend you eat curries! Just don't pig on the carbs that tend to go with it!

Note: try to get good quality organic turmeric; what you find in the supermarket is pretty variable and likely accompanied by manufacturing excipients, such as magnesium stearate.

Caralluma fimbrata

Also known as: C. Fimbriate, Caraluma, Caralluma ascendens, Caralluma Cactus, Caralluma Extract, Caralluma fimbriata, Caralluma Fimbriata Extract, Caraluma Pregnane Glycosides.

Native tribespeople and nomads carried this plant with them, for use in times of hunger. They call it a "famine food," because when food is scarce, you can kill off your appetite and get by when there's not much to live on... Apparently, hunters could last for a week on this plant alone.

Developing evidence suggests that pregnane glycosides are the magical ingredient and taking a Caralluma extract for 60 days might decrease waistline, feelings of hunger, and fat and calorie intake. In the medical journal *Appetite*, researchers reported that when they studied this food, people lost inches around their waist and their appetite was lessened. But it does not seem to decrease weight, body mass index (BMI), body fat, or hip measurements. [7]

Caralluma seems to be safe for most people when 500 mg of the extract is taken twice daily for up to 60 days. The long-term safety effects are not known, according to WebMD, so don't take it for longer.[8]

Hoodia

Hoodia enjoys a less than salubrious reputation, undoubtedly due to overarching marketing claims and methods. But essentially, it is the same as Caralluma, meaning its effect is based around pregnane glycosides.

Hoodia gordonii is a succulent plant native to South Africa and Asia where indigenous populations have traditionally used it, most notably the Khoi-San, as an appetite and thirst suppressant during long hunting expeditions into harsh environments.

Like Caralluma, Hoodia acts by curbing hunger; it tricks your brain into believing that you are full and it will not signal hunger pangs. The laboratory evidence for this assertion was produced by David MacLean, MD, an adjunct associate professor at Brown University, and a former researcher at the pharmaceutical giant, Pfizer. In a report published in the Sept. 10, 2004, issue of *Brain Research*, MacLean reported that a molecule in hoodia, called P57, likely has an effect on the brain's hypothalamus, which helps regulate appetite. However, his study was done entirely with animals. [9]

Phytopharm, a UK-based company developing hoodia weight loss products with Unilever, the giant food and consumer products company, cites its own 2001 study on its website, in which the plant extract caused a reduction in average daily calorie intake and in body fat within two weeks. Caloric intake dropped by about 1,000 a day after about two weeks, according to the study. (Phytopharm was originally developing P57 with Pfizer, but Pfizer returned its rights to Phytopharm in 2003.)

In other words, the hoodia science is sketchy but believable. The bottom line here seems more to do with the authenticity of the product, than any real concern if it works: there's plenty of fake hoodia being sold. Most products don't have enough hoodia in them to work. Best avoided for that reason.[10]

Sacred Lotus (Nelumbo nucifera)

Also known as Indian lotus, sacred lotus, bean of India, or simply lotus.

The flowers, seeds, young leaves, and roots are all edible but should not be eaten raw; there is a risk of parasite transmission (e.g., Fasciolopsis buski). In Asia, the petals are sometimes used for garnish, while the large leaves are used as a wrap for food. In Korea and Vietnam it is used as a tea infusion.

Young lotus stems are used as a salad ingredient in Vietnamese cuisine. The rhizome and the roots are used as a vegetable in soups, deep-fried, stir-fried, and braised dishes.

Lotus rootlets are often pickled with rice vinegar, sugar, chili and/or garlic. It has a crunchy texture with sweet-tangy flavors. In Asian cuisine, it is popular with salad, prawns, sesame oil and/or coriander leaves.

Lotus roots have been found to be rich in dietary fiber, vitamin C, potassium, thiamin, riboflavin, vitamin B6, phosphorus, copper, and manganese, while very low in saturated fat and. [11]

An article in the *American Journal of Botany* reported that lotus seeds 1,300 years old were able to germinate successfully, so maybe this venerable plant has a lot to teach us about health and longevity. Part of that is weight control. [12]

In a study published in the *Journal of Ethnopharmacology*, the Sacred Lotus prevented the increase in body weight, and promoted the breakdown of fat in adipose tissue in animals [13]

Beware The Scams

That's about as far as the meaningful science goes. Beware the marketing of products with phoney science, that's dressed up to look real. It's no big deal or big expense to pay some shill scientist or doctor to run a short series as a "study" and publish the trial in a journal that sounds respectable. Remember, journals are often struggling for funding and someone who pays for a series of ads is a very attractive "customer" and is likely to get favorable editorial space (indeed, on a massive scale, this is exactly why drug company science gets published, even when it's of a very poor standard).

Many so-called clinical trials are carried out in poorer countries, with ethical standards easily corrupted by the promise of even a little money. Take for example the green coffee bean story. Suddenly, green coffee bean extract was a wonder weight loss miracle; it was featured by Dr. Mehmet Oz on US TV.

What was shown as clinical "proof" was a very sub-standard trial, with only 16 cases, carried out in India by a team under Joe Vinson, a chemist at the University of Scranton, Pennsylvania. It was paid for by the supplement manufacturer Applied Food Sciences in Texas, which is always a red flag, and published in the online journal Diabetes, Metabolic Syndrome and Obesity: Targets and Therapy. This trial was never pre-registered, a standard requirement these days, so negative results cannot be simply buried.

This study has some serious methodological problems including the small sample size, lack of proper blinding, doses, unreliable diet recalls, and repeated measurements. In short, it is more or less junk science. But the word of a medical TV celebrity like Dr. Oz can set off a storm of sales and that's what happened.

See earlier this section for a note on green coffee bean extract, combined with Garcinia cambogia.

Sensa "Diet"

While on the subject of phoney science, dressed up as real fact, check this product out. If B*S* was digestible, you could probably sustain yourself for months on Sensa "Sprinkles".

Alan Hirsch, MD, founder and neurologic director of the Smell and Taste Treatment and Research Foundation in Chicago, developed Sensa crystals or "tastants" that promote feelings of fullness and, ultimately, weight loss. If you stick with Sensa, the promotional blurb says you could lose 30 pounds in six months. Yeah, right.

Of course anyone could lose 30 pounds in six months. I did it in only 5 weeks after my first wife left! (Couldn't face food). All you have to do to lose 30 pounds is just eat less! You don't need fancy crystals.

There is nothing unique about the list of ingredients in Sensa food flakes. They are made from maltodextrin, tricalcium phosphate, caramine, FD&C Yellow 5, silica, natural and artificial flavors, soy, and milk ingredients. A no-no then for dairy allergics, anyway.

There is no MSG. But maltodextrin is one of the dreaded corn sugars family and something no human should eat by choice.

You sprinkle Sensa flakes on food as you would salt or sugar, and they enhance scent while adding either a mildly salty or sweet taste. Savory flavors include cheddar cheese, onion, horseradish, ranch dressing, taco, and Parmesan cheese. Sweet flavors are cocoa, spearmint, banana, strawberry, raspberry, and malt.

All the tastants it is claimed are calorie-free, sugar-free, sodium-free, and gluten-free. Well of course! They are food-free as well! It's all chemicals, sugar, dyes and artificial flavors. Don't think the onion sprinkles have onion, it's "onion flavor".

Only an American would come up with the absurd idea that to get the taste of good food, you have to fake it and make it. The rest of us, if we accept the hypothesis that the taste of good food is enough to make us eat less, we choose good FOOD!

Hirsch uses the term "sensory-specific satiety" to describe the process by which smell receptors send messages of fullness to your brain. Sounds good but there's not a shred of meaningful science; just lots of bogus testimonials. For example when I went to the website a woman called Gaylene was featured, who claimed to have lost 62 lbs in 18 months.

But then it also says Gaylene was paid for saying this! (compensated for excellent results is the actual wording). Plus it says she followed a sensible diet for 18 months. Great! So she didn't need the Sensa product at all. [14]

A one-month Sensa starter kit costing $59, and a 6-month kit at an introductory rate of $235, are available on the Sensa web site. There's also a "free trial", with the usual trickery, so that you end up giving them your credit card details and YOU are then supposed to cancel. If you don't, you'll be charged. Plus the refund is mailed at your own expense and you don't qualify unless you send all of the product back within 30 days. How can you? You've opened the packet and tried it!

What's the Science?

Pitiful. Just a few "clinical studies" by Hirsch himself. These were in no way clinical trials. These studies have not been published in a peer-reviewed medical journal.

In an independent investigation, ABC News found that the participants of the study were not weighed in by the researchers, but instead weighed themselves at home with no outside verification.

Moreover, it turns out that many of the participants were doing other weight loss regimes at the same time, so it is quite possible, even probable, the users who lost weight did so for entirely another reason than the Sensa flakes.

Hirsch acknowledged that his promotional videos falsely claimed that the study used "placebo" flakes on a control group to simulate Sensa flakes. It did not. So Hirsch is dishonest. That's bad. Why would you buy his product anyway?

The Federal Trade Commission finally took action against the Sensa marketing company, stating that its ads were misleading. In January 2014, Sensa agreed to pay $26.5 million to settle the FTC's charges.

Sensa is still selling its products. "Sensa's safety is not an issue," the company's web site states.

Sensa notes that it "has agreed to make changes to its advertising claims" and hasn't admitted any wrongful conduct. Well, liars never do own up, do they?

Not Such A Good Idea (Ephedra)

Ephedra is an herb. It has been banned in the U.S., ostensibly due to safety concerns. Mormon tea and ephedra are sometimes confused. Mormon tea or American ephedra comes from Ephedra nevadensis, it does not contain ephedrine and so does not give the buzz or pop; the weightloss drug ephedra (also known as ma huang) comes primarily from the plant *Ephedra sinica* and because it contains ephedrine, there are potentially serious side effects.

In addition to its use for weight loss and obesity and to enhance athletic performance, Ephedra is also used for allergies and hay fever; nasal congestion; and respiratory tract conditions such as bronchospasm, asthma, and bronchitis. It has been used for colds, flu, swine flu, fever, chills, headache, inability to sweat, joint and bone pain, and as a "water pill" to increase urine flow in people who retain fluids.

On December 30, 2003, the FDA announced the ban of ephedra products in the U.S., effective April 2004. The FDA claimed that ephedra raises blood pressure, stresses the circulatory system and "poses an unreasonable risk" to the health of people who take ephedra weight loss products.

In April 2005, the dietary supplement industry successfully challenged the FDA ban on ephedra. A year after the ban on ephedra began, a federal judge in Utah struck down the FDA's action saying that

FDA didn't prove that low doses of ephedra are harmful. In August 2006, an appeal court reversed the Utah judge's decision and upheld the FDA's ban of ephedra-containing dietary supplements.

The truth is Ephedra contains a chemical called ephedrine, which stimulates the heart, the lungs, and the nervous system. In addition, it can cause tremors, anxiety attacks and even psychotic episodes; kidney stones; rapid heart rate and increased blood pressure; tension, flushing and sweating; lack of sleep (bad); loss of appetite (good).

The risk of side effects and adverse effects appears to be greater in people with preexisting conditions, such as heart disease, high blood pressure; heart rate disorders; thyroid disease; hypoglycemia; glaucoma; diabetes; kidney disease or kidney stones; anxiety disorder; mental illness or a history of mental illness; enlarged prostate; cerebral insufficiency and a history of seizures, stroke, or transient ischemic attacks. People with allergies to ephedra, ephedrine, or pseudoephedrine should avoid ephedra. If in doubt, consult with your primary care physician.

All in all, this is one for everyone to avoid. Don't let the marketers get to you, even if Ephedra is legal in your territory.

Bitter Orange

Because the sale of ephedra weight loss pills remains illegal, the weight loss supplement industry has begun marketing "ephedra-free," "ephedrine-free" or "legal" ephedra products, in which ephedra is replaced with other weight loss stimulants, like bitter orange and caffeine.

However, bitter orange contains chemicals similar to ephedra, such as synephrine and octopamine, which may speed up your heart rate and increase your blood pressure, so bitter orange is not a safe replacement for ephedra weight loss supplements.

If you wanted to lose weight, you might have been tempted to try Slimming Beauty Bitter Orange Slimming Capsules, a weight loss dietary supplement sold on the Internet. The label claimed that Slimming Beauty was "100% herbal" and "a natural vitamin and calcium" capsule for use even by children as young as two. But the label didn't have two important warnings: First, that Slimming Beauty was illegally spiked with dangerous amounts of sibutramine, a powerful prescription-strength stimulant. Second, if you had tried it, you could have had a heart attack.

If the word sibutramine sounds familiar, that's because it's the generic name for Meridia, the prescription weight loss drug withdrawn from the market in October 2010, at the FDA's request.

Though the agency had approved the drug in 1997, a recent 10,000-patient, 6-year study showed that sibutramine upped the risk of nonfatal "cardiovascular events" like heart attacks and strokes by 16%, causing the FDA to reconsider.

In other words the suppliers of Slimming Beauty were liars and fakers, claiming "natural" and "100% herbal". This is more than crime; it's risking murder or at the very least manslaughter.

Just be careful what you take and stay within these guidelines. Know that one study by the US Mayo Clinic found diet pills containing caffeine and bitter orange extract together were linked to increased blood pressure, strokes and heart attacks.

Yohimbine is another "natural" herbal stimulant that can cause side effects, such as rapid heart rate, high blood pressure, headaches and has even been linked to heart attack, seizures and kidney failure.

Beware That "All Natural" Label!

Dishonest and sleazy merchants often use the term "all natural" on their supplement labels; not because their product is in any way natural but because they find that this description sells more product! People want to believe that what they are getting is good, natural and wholesome and so they make their choices with this in mind. It's easy to sucker trusting and caring people into believing they are doing the right thing.

In recent years, the FDA tested the contents of many weight loss supplements touted as "all natural." The agency found that nearly 70 of those supplements contained ingredients such as:

- controlled substances
- seizure medications
- prescription drugs

In recent years, the FDA has gone after more than 70 tainted weight loss products, many with names like Slim Burn, 24 Hours Diet, and Natural Model, after finding that they had been adulterated with undeclared stimulants, diuretics, and even antidepressants, often in amounts exceeding the maximum recommended dosages at which such drugs can be safely prescribed.

Because of the uncertainty of the ingredients in weight loss supplements, it is strongly recommended that you talk to your health care provider before trying them.

You should also check with your health care provider to make sure the supplement you're considering will not interact with other medications you are taking.

The Cinnamon Scam

You've probably heard that the common kitchen spice cinnamon can have a positive impact on your insulin sensitivity, allowing your body to better process the carbohydrates you eat. Insulin sensitivity means better blood sugar control, weight loss and greater health for you (see section 8).

The most fragrant and delicate cinnamon (the real deal) is obtained from the *Cinnamomum zeylanicum* a tree native to Sri Lanka (which used to be called 'Ceylon' or Zeylan in Latin), the Malabar coast of India and Myanmar (Burma). This cinnamon is sometimes called 'true cinnamon' or 'old-fashioned cinnamon.'

But here's something you may not know... that cinnamon that you have in your kitchen cupboard is probably not cinnamon at all if you bought it at the grocery store. Online, the story is probably even worse; there is no real way to tell.

Believe it or not, out of 12 samples of ground cinnamon examined by the New York Board of Health, *only three contained any cinnamon whatsoever* and even those were largely mixed with sawdust. The others were almost entirely composed of sawdust, starch, and cinnamon flavored oil.

Beyond that, most cinnamon that you find at the grocery store, even if genuine, has been heavily irradiated to extend its shelf life. This irradiation process destroys many of the active nutrients found in cinnamon, thus inactivating its ability to produce any health-promoting benefits.

Another common problem is that what is being sold as cinnamon is actually Cassia or "Chinese cinnamon", from the *Cinnamomum cassia* tree (a lot of which is now grown in northern Vietnam and exported from there). We don't have the same science for Cassia yet.

To be sure you are getting proper cinnamon, the real spice, best buy the sticks and powder them yourself, using a blender or grinder.

What About That Carb Neutralizer?

It's called the "carb neutralizer" or "starch blocker". To read the manufacturer's and marketer's blurb, you would think it's a cinch: all you have to do is take this supplement and you are good. The pounds will melt off.

Their science says this stuff stops the digestion of starches and therefore they are not available, metabolically, from your food. Bingo! You lose weight quickly and easily.

So what is this wonder supplement? White kidney beans... *Phaseolus vulgaris*. The idea doesn't impress me but... where there is a dollar to be made, there you will find the eager marketers, beavering away to try and persuade you that, without their goods, you haven't a chance of getting what you want.

It may be strong to call this supplement a scam... but kidney beans? I mean, come on. Eat a good chilli con carne!

Makers say that by blocking a starch-digesting enzyme called alpha-amylase, these carb neutralizers or starch blockers prevent the body from absorbing carbs—sparing you from the carb calories. I'm not big on blocking a body process that Nature put there for us. How can we know that's safe?

Starch blockers are dietary supplements, not prescription drugs. Since they don't go through the FDA's drug approval process, the FDA has not signed-off on whether starch blockers are safe, effective, or contain what the label says is in the bottle.

Trouble is, even if the starch blockers do allow complex carbohydrates to pass through the small intestine largely undigested, there's eventual trouble. When the unprocessed foods get to the large intestine, the starches ferment, give off gas ("blowing off" or farting), and cause bloating and diarrhea, also a somewhat unpleasant side effect.

Not recommended. Just eat less carbs, for Heaven's sake!

That "WeightLoss4Idiots" Scam

Now a doctor, a Georgia chiropractor named Suzanne Gudakunst, has apparently angered Big Pharma, the medical industry, as well as food companies that manufacture weight loss supplements and food products because of what she claims is a breakthrough secret: a parasite cleanse (see section 13). She's getting death threats, she says (but that could be a clever marketing ploy; hold on).

Turns out the this Suzanne Gudakunst is the person who foisted the "FatLoss4Idiots" program on the unsuspecting public, now called the "FatLossSecret", all marketed via the Internet, with outrageous claims not backed up by any credible science.

Trouble is, if you go online for a "review" of such products and their claims, you can't trust what you read. Everybody is supporting everybody else with lies, because they are all "affiliates", in on the money.

Every one of these eager beavers posters of "reviews" has an affiliate link to the sales page, meaning he or she gets paid if you buy.

Doc Susie, you might want to take a look at some of the claims your affiliates are making. Such as this gem...

"So powerful is her secret that she's able to reverse diabetes, rid illness altogether in people suffering from cancer (linked directly to poor diet and overweight factors), as well as an elimination of an entire spectrum of serious and otherwise life-threatening diseases."

What is this amazing "secret" weight loss cure, that almost got her murdered by enraged competitors? You'll laugh!

1. psyllium husks fiber or oat bran fiber
2. milk thistle seed extract
3. herbal laxatives: cascara sagrada bark and senna leaf
4. anti-parasite herbal remedy: black walnut hulls, wormwood, and cloves.

All these remedies do work in their way but there is nothing new here and nothing special about this formula, much less unique. Don't fall for the marketing hype.

You can learn about these remedies anywhere, without paying the mysterious "Doctor" Suzanne Gudakunst a hefty $57.

Caveat emptor is my advice.

Do Weight Loss Pills Have A Place?

Don't forget the term "slimming pills" may be taken to include proprietary mixtures, as well as prescription medication. There can be considerable dangers to taking unregulated formulas and, it has to be said, women have died. You don't want to put your life at risk, in your desperation to lose weight.

Better fat than dead, to paraphrase a famous 60s quote from philosopher Bertrand Russell!

The danger really starts when you go on the Internet to find quick solution to weight issues. It's always risky to generalize but there are vast numbers of dishonest promoters out there, who want your money and don't really care what happens to you.

The lovely glowing stories of the successful cases they claim are almost always false or, if not, then it's just a lucky one or two out of hundreds or thousands.

In an article dated 18 July 2013, the British newspaper *The Daily Mail* carried an article with dire reports of the possible dangers of ordering unknown and unregulated products from an online source.

One 19 year old woman, wanting to lose weight fast, had tried a host of diets from Atkins to Weight Watchers with no apparent success. Then, with the help of misguided friends, she found a product on eBay called Grenade Fat Burner, and it didn't take her long to find a variety of "Pink Grenades" for sale on eBay for around £35 a tub.

She saw the word herbal and thought that meant "safe". All she really cared about then was whether they helped her lose weight – which they did straight away. She carried on taking them on holiday and came back two sizes smaller. She never felt hungry and only wanted to eat a third of her normal portion size at each meal. In less than six months, she'd dropped over 50 pounds and dropped three dress sizes. It was as if she'd had a gastric band fitted!

She was so delighted with the weight she lost from her eBay-bought pills that she continued taking them on and off for three years – ignoring the frequent headaches, her racing heart rate at night and the constant cystitis that she had begun to suffer from.

What this lady didn't know at the time was that these pills (since reformulated) contained stimulants and appetite suppressants that have been linked to a range of health problems, especially including bladder troubles and heart attacks.

So the final cost of fast weight loss was horrendous. She may never be healthy again.

The UK's Medicines and Healthcare Products Regulatory Agency, or MHRA, admits the problem is enormous and in June 2013 seized a record £12 million worth of fake and unlicensed medicine—much of it slimming pills.

The MHRA also shut down 1,300 UK-based websites selling the drugs online.

Of the vast array of legal and illegal diet pills available online, many are simply ineffectual and a waste of money. But others are potentially fatal as they contain prescription-only or banned ingredients.

Definitely Dangerous

The same newspapers reported a 20-year-old girl who suffered a fatal heart attack after overdosing on 20 slimming pills containing the stimulant DMAA, which gave her a caffeine hit equivalent to drinking 40 cups of coffee.

DMAA (dimethylamylamine or 1,3-amphetamine or simply dimethylamylamine), is not illegal to take or possess in the UK, but is not licensed, so, in theory, it shouldn't be sold. However it's easy enough to purchase online.

In another tragedy, a 23-year-old medical student who had a history of eating disorders, was found dead in bed by flatmates after taking a fatal dose of a slimming pill called DNP, which she'd bought online.

DNP is a pesticide banned for human consumption but openly sold on the internet as a quick-fix weight-loss pill – one of its side effects is that it causes a rise in body temperature and in large doses can cause death by literally cooking the body from within.

My point is that it takes the enaction of a law to get these money-making medical thugs to stop hurting people. Their greed is such that they don't care who they hurt, so long as they get rich peddling suspect and dangerous wares.

There's the added complication of some companies exploiting legal loopholes by marketing pills with clever wording, or selling via third parties on sites such as eBay, making the real seller hard to trace.

Don't fall for it. As I urge you all through this book, the real path to effective and lifelong weight control is education and working along with nature, not trying to take sleazy short cuts. There are no real short cuts to weight loss; only to the mortuary.

Always consult with a knowledgeable healthcare practitioner for advice on weight loss medications. Proper prescription drugs will be quite safe, right? Wrong. Those are just as bad or worse.

Read on...

Pharmaceutical Drugs Dangerous Too

Pharmaceutical weight control drugs are mainly toxic and of uncertain action. The rush to get them to the market and start making money leads to constant violation of safety procedures. To use such a heavy chemical bombardment on the body to get such a trivial result as loss of appetite is an abuse in my opinion, notwithstanding the possible very serious consequences of overweight and obesity.

If you don't share my cynicism, look at the history of the pharmaceutical industry. Many of today's leading companies are members of the German cartel IG Farben, which built its might on the use of slave labor in Nazi concentration camps (a bit different to proper commercial achievement, don't you think?)

These pharmaceutical companies include BASF, Bayer, Hoechst, and other German chemical and pharmaceutical companies. IG Farben was the single largest donor to the election campaign of Adolph Hitler. One year before Hitler seized power, IG Farben donated 400,000 marks to Hitler and his Nazi party.

The Nazis are gone, but not the crimes against humanity. Merck, the company that Hitler personally invested in, has one of the worst records in modern times. With a long list of deaths to its credit, and more than $5.5 billion in judgments and fines levied against it, it was five years before Merck made its $30-billion recall of the painkiller Vioxx. After the drug was withdrawn, and 60,000 had already died, Merck picked up the pieces painlessly by getting a new drug fast-tracked and on the market.

Good old Bayer released the nicotinoid chemicals that may have killed off millions of bees. Are they sorry? No, the first reaction of these greedy corporate thugs is to sue the European Commission to overturn a ban on their dangerous pesticides.

Bayer and Syngenta, two of the world's largest chemical corporations, claim that the ban is "unjustified" and "disproportionate." But clear scientific evidence shows their products are behind the massive bee die-off that puts our entire food chain in peril.

So you are not going to find me recommending products from these twisted and destructive companies. That said, I promised you an overview of all the information about weight loss. In order to fulfill that undertaking, I am entering a section here to look at their offerings.

Weight Loss Medicines Reviewed

In my younger days, Ponderax (fenfluramine) was the thing, or it's relative Adifax (dexfenfluramine). These drugs were supposed to suppress appetite. But both substances were taken off the market in 1997 because they tend to cause progressive damage to heart valves (If you took either of these weight loss medications for three months or more, it would be a good idea to see a doctor and get tested).

But even before that, there were concerns about the amphetamine-like nature of such compounds. People taking them became aroused, over-stimulated, restless, tense and anxious. That's what amphetamines do to a person and why amphetamines and similar substances are government regulated.

Still the idea persists in the pharmaceutical industry: that there is a lot of profit to be made in the slimming market and an effective appetite suppressant would be a real money-spinner. When sales are in the offing, the industry has shown itself to be very lacking in scruples over safety matters. And so it remains with appetite suppressants.

Current synthetic offerings, like mazindol, phentermine, benzphetamine and diethylpropion, cause numerous amphetamine-like side effects, such as nervousness, palpitations, tremors (shaking of the hands), restlessness, high blood pressure and insomnia. Other undesirable effects include sweating, excessive thirst and constipation. Ironically, while appetite suppressants can keep you awake, they can also cause drowsiness. Overdose levels can lead to confusion, convulsions or seizures, hallucinations, and even coma.

On no account allow yourself to take one of these drugs, even if prescribed by a physician, if any of the following conditions apply: pregnancy, breastfeeding, allergies, diabetes, hypertension, kidney disease, heart disease, seizures or epilepsy, glaucoma, hyperthyroidism (overactive thyroid), mental disturbance, or a history of abuse of alcohol or drugs.

Moreover, these substances can be dangerous in the presence of many other drugs, because they can alter the way your body eliminates the drug and predispose you to side effects. Just don't take them!

The Orlistat Family

Another type of prescription weight loss drug is a fat absorption inhibitor. They work by preventing your body from breaking down and absorbing fats eaten with your meals. This unabsorbed fat is eliminated in bowel movements. Orlistat is the only drug of this type in the U.S. It is available by prescription as Xenical and over-the-counter as Alli, a reduced-strength version.

At the standard prescription dose of 120 mg three times daily before meals, Orlistat prevents approximately 30% of dietary fat from being absorbed and about 25% in the standard over-the- counter dose of 60 mg. Higher doses do not produce more potent effects. [15]

Well, that's pretty stupid all by itself. We need fats to be healthy and process our vitamins. Some fats, indeed, are essential: so-called essential fatty acids or EFAs (omega-3s and omega-6s). Our brains are rich in fats. How is blocking fat absorption going to help strengthen and maintain our brain tissue?

The most obvious and unpleasant side-effect of this type of drug is fecal incontinence, meaning the person poops his or her pants. It's not that sphincter muscles fail (real incontinence) but that the urge to pass feces comes on so suddenly that the person can't stop the urge. You may know, there have been embarrassing disasters in which someone lets rip in the swimming pool or jacuzzi.

The effectiveness of Orlistat in promoting weight loss is definite, though unimpressive. Pooled data from clinical trials suggest that people given Orlistat in addition to lifestyle modifications, such as diet and exercise, lose about 2–3 kilograms (5 - 6 lbs.) more than those not taking the drug over the course of a year. [16]

I don't think the unpleasantness makes Orlistat justified, for a mere 6 lbs. a year. Undoubtedly the poor effect is due to the fact that carbohydrates are the real problem, not fats, as is commonly supposed. Moreover there have been no real safety studies, therefore its over-the-counter status is highly improper.

All I can say is a big proportion of our vital nutrients are fat soluble, meaning if we reduce fat intake, we get less of these important nutrients. I'm thinking of vitamins A, D, E and K, for example.

Other prescription weight loss pills, like Adipex-P, are approved only for short-term use (usually 12 weeks or less) and have not been studied for their long-term effectiveness.

Unsafe Strategies With Drugs

In their desperation to achieve effective weight loss, some people are resorting to ridiculous, even dangerous procedures, and you should not put yourself at risk by trying to emulate them.

Here are some notes...

Laxatives And Purges

Purging is definitely NOT recommended for weight loss. By purging I mean making yourself vomit, chewing food and spitting it out, and/or abusing laxatives. It's what silly girls who end up with anorexia/bulimia get up to: eat food and then make their body give it up, either through vomiting it back or diarrhea and purges. These unhealthy and unsafe behaviors are not uncommon on college campuses, pose serious health problems, and are the first step in the development of eating disorders.

For one thing, acid in the stomach is extremely strong. Strong acid is necessary to prepare food for digestion and extremely acidic vomit can cause erosion in the esophagus and mouth and damage tooth enamel.

Regular purging by vomiting or abuse of laxatives also causes excess fluid loss that can cause serious dehydration and electrolyte imbalances.

One particularly dangerous purge is syrup of Ipecac; one dose can trigger cardiac irregularity and can lead to cardiac arrest.

Experts even say this can increase risk for certain cancers.

Tobacco Use

Despite decades of awareness of the countless health risks of tobacco, some people—especially young adults—turn to smoking as a diet strategy.

Everyone knows that smokers, when they quit, tend to pile on the weight. It's true that nicotine is an appetite suppressant, but the risks of smoking cigarettes vastly outweigh any supposed benefits.

Smoking harms nearly every organ of the body; causes cancer as well as cardiovascular, respiratory, and other diseases; reduces the health of smokers in general; and increases the risk of death.

This sounds like a list of problems caused by obesity too. Well, one is as bad as the other.

But there is one logical reason not to use smoking for weight loss, beyond the numerous health risks, which is that weight gain is often a side effect when the smoker later tries to kick the addictive habit. You could become trapped by your own solution.

Don't smoke for any reason, least of all to lose weight.

Abusing Drugs

Quite apart from the inherent dangers in medically licensed drugs for weight loss that I have described here, there is the issue of abuse of drugs. Using street drugs or inappropriate medications for weight loss is a grim mistake and fraught with all kinds of consequences. It could cost you your health, your happiness and even your life.

The real dangers of abusing cocaine, speed, and meds such as those prescribed for attention deficit disorder (Ritalin or Adderall), thyroid disorders, or diabetes to lose weight, far outweigh any health benefit you may get from weight loss. Just some of the unintended risks include, physical and psychological addiction, social and financial problems (these substances cost money), anxiety, severe headaches, stroke, and heart, lung, and kidney damage.

For example, DXM, or dextromethorphan, is a common ingredient in cough and combination cold medicines. Teens exploit it for highs. DXM is in almost half of all of the OTC drugs sold in the US, making it cheap, easy to get, and legal.

A 2008 study found that one in 10 American teenagers has abused products with DXM, making it more popular in that age group than cocaine, ecstasy, LSD, and methamphetamine.

One of the pronounced effects of DXM is weight loss and youngsters concerned about their weight may be tempted to try it. Don't even think about this kind of folly. Such a short cut to weight loss may be a short cut to the grave, as I said.

Using illegal drugs for any purpose is strongly discouraged, and using legal drugs for any unintended purpose without medical supervision is just as dangerous.

PART 2. THE ISSUES

SECTION 11. ENDOCRINE FACTORS IN WEIGHT CONTROL

You've heard people say, "It's my glands; whatever I eat goes onto my waist." Well, it might just be true; at least for some people.

The one gland that does majorly control metabolic rate and body weight is the thyroid gland. When its function deteriorates, weight gain is an inevitable concomitant, yet thyroid problems are rarely diagnosed, because laboratory results come back "normal".

Technically, weight gain due to low thyroid is of special character and is called myxedema: the skin is puffy (edema), but there is also fatigue, depression, sensitivity to cold, swellings, dry skin, brittle hair that falls out, heavy menses (women), late or absent periods, low blood pressure, shortness of breath, slow speech, lethargy and even seizures.

Why is it so under-diagnosed? Because doctors rely too much on blood tests and, in this case, a blood test which is all but worthless (TSH). Not that it's inaccurate; but orthodox interpretation of what it means is way off target.

Good holistic doctors will follow the symptoms and treat the clinical condition, which clearly exists. The fact is that up to 20% of the population is probably suffering from some degree of hypothyroidism (low thyroid function), though in some territories it could be much higher. The older you get, the more prone you are to the condition; it's part of natural ageing. But it is still pathological and it should be treated!

But if the TSH result is "normal", conventional doctors declare there is no problem and the thyroid is fine. They say this even when there are striking symptoms, such as fatigue, slowed speech, depression, weight-gain, dry skin, hair loss and other easily visible signs of low thyroid function. How crazy is it to state to a patient that, "We have done all the tests and there is nothing wrong," when the patient says she feels awful?

Part of the problem is that the usually quoted lab ranges are so wide that measurements are relatively meaningless and you could be 50% down on average and still said to be within "normal" limits.

The real point is that a person can be functionally and clinically hypothyroid without any abnormal blood markers. It's a test of a doctor's skill to recognize and treat the disease they see, whether or not the laboratory is helpful in confirming the diagnosis.

It is vital that all doctors start to think more often of thyroid problems. Because it's not just an overweight or "quality of life" issue: your risk of heart disease is significantly increased and the confusion and lethargy which comes on may even be mistaken for senility and the patient put on a completely inappropriate program.

Plus, we all live in an iodine-starved world and iodine is a vital fuel that is needed for correct thyroid functioning. Yes, they add iodine to table salt (not much!) but then they put bromine in bread and other foods, which directly inhibits the availability of iodine.

Trust me, YOU are short of iodine. We all are. Yet it's not often prescribed and difficult to get hold of. You need to add it to your supplements right now.

The most potent form is called Lugol's iodine, a mixture of iodine and potassium iodide. Professor Guy Abraham has developed Lugol's iodine into a tablet form (Iodoral) which is well tolerated. It contains a mixture of 5mg of iodine and 7.5mg of iodide. He recommends a three month loading dose of 4 tablets daily, starting off with 1 tablet a day for a week, then 2 tablets daily for a week, 3 tablets daily for a week and then 4 tablets.

After three months the dose should then be reduced to a maintenance dose of 1 tablet daily. You could be surprised by the weight benefits, just from the one simple strategy. You may also notice a definite increase in wellbeing and energy levels, with lessening brain fog.

You can buy Iodoral on Amazon, at the time of writing.

Thyroiditis

Women have a high incidence of a clinical condition called Hashimoto's disease (auto-immune thyroiditis), in which the body makes antibodies against its own thyroid gland and hormones. It's one of those allergy-against-yourself diseases (rheumatoid arthritis is another).

It must be mentioned in passing that there is another kind of thyroiditis. This is not caused by anti-bodies but a virus, typically mumps or Coxsackie. Usually it resolves clinically but may be the source of chronic hypothyroidism.

Pioneer, the late Dr Broda O. Barnes, a US physician, reckoned that hypothyroidism underpinned a huge range of diseases in the West, from heart disease, to allergies; cancer to apparent parasitism; loss of sexual function to poor visual acuity. Notice, by the way, how those are like a catalogue of aging problems!

But it's not just about pseudo-aging: for women, all kinds of menstrual difficulties—notably heavy flow—can be attributed to hypothyroidism, as can emotional and behavioral problems in children. Indeed, there is a clear link between hypothyroidism and autism spectrum disorder.

Of course what we are most interested in for this text is relentless and uncontrollable weight gain. If thyroid is the problem, it has to be uncovered and properly solved.

But I am giving you the wider picture, because seeing other related symptoms and conditions may enable you to spot the problem, when others around you are not seeing it.

If you suspect a thyroid problem may be the cause of your weight worries, what can you do? There is a very simple, convenient test that you can do for yourself, which is almost 100% reliable to detecting a low thyroid problem. It was discovered by Dr. Broda Barnes MD.

The Broda Barnes Temperature Test

A simple test for thyroid function, which can be very revealing, is to take regular morning measurements of basal *temperature.*

Basal temperature means while at absolute rest. In ordinary terms that means first thing on waking, after the body has been lying still overnight. Temperature drops to its lowest at this point. To measure your own basal temperature, use a clinical thermometer, keep it in your armpit (or rectally, if you've a mind), before getting out of bed or any activity whatsoever. Wait at least 10 minutes (3 minutes rectally). Record the results.

You probably know that the average temperature of an adult with a healthy thyroid and a healthy metabolism is 98.6 degrees Fahrenheit or 37.0 degrees Celsius, and that occurs around mid- afternoon.

Generally, if the waking temperature in the armpit is running at less than 97.8, that is presumptive evidence of low thyroid function (rectal temperature should be at least 98.2).

Allowance may need to be made for women who are ovulating, since the temperature naturally rises about 0.5 of a degree at this time.

Treatment

I might point out that it's becoming increasingly dangerous for a qualified doctor to treat thyroid problems naturally and doctors have had their license rescinded for treating patients with "normal" thyroid labs.

In my UK practice I used a several-fold approach. The simplest, if the signs are early enough and the patient is otherwise vigorous, is homeopathic thyroid stimulant. I used a product called *Thyroidea compositum* from Germany. It is one of the most powerful and useful non-drug substances a doctor can have in his or her repertoire. Such is its impact of the thyroid on immunity, that I found myself also prescribing this compound often for my cancer patients seeking alternative remedies.

If a trial of this substance and related compounds appears ineffective, then supplementation with the hormone can be considered. Conventional colleagues would not normally approach things this way, feeling that if the blood levels are "adequate" then supplementation is pointless.

The stupidity of this attitude is that they then have nothing to offer the patient, beyond palliative treatment. Often this means prescribing anti-depressants for the lethargy or depression and giving him or her a good ticking off about being overweight!

A better approach is to use what we call a "therapeutic trial". The patient then becomes his or her own test bed. If taking the hormone results in a rapid return to normal, with renewed zest and loss of weight encumbrance, is that not adequate intellectual evidence that the thyroid was indeed, in some way, under-performing?

Synthetic vs. Natural Replacement

The usual thyroid hormone Synthroid (levothyroxine) is synthetically produced. There are considerations that make the natural product better. This means supplementing dried (desiccated) thyroid extract from animal sources (pig instead of beef, because of BSE). But if Hashimoto's disease is the problem, synthetic products may occasionally be better, because the body doesn't react to them in the same way.

Animal thyroid extract has been on the market and safely used for more than 100 years. When synthetic thyroxine was introduced, there was a great deal of baloney and marketing hype about how modern it was, compared to "old-fashioned" desiccated thyroid—and many doctors switched patients over to the synthetic medication. When the patient went into a steep decline as a result, he or she was told, "It's your age."

The best-known natural desiccated thyroid extract is Armour. Other brand names include Nature-throid, and Westhroid.

All along, Synthroid has been sponsor of medical meetings, golf outings, symposia, research grants, and speakers' fees, and is the chief provider of lunches at medical offices, patient literature, pens, pads, mugs, and other freebies, giveaways, and marketing items for decades.

As a result, we now have several generations of doctors who have been trained to believe that synthetic levothyroxine, and specifically Synthroid, is the only thyroid replacement medication available or worth using. They simply don't know anything else. They hear ridiculous rumors on a regular basis, spread by drug reps for competitive levothyroxine drugs, that desiccated thyroid is going off the market.

Pseudo-Science and Hype

Most doctors claim their opposition to desiccated thyroid is science-based. However, that's not true, because there are no double-blind, peer-reviewed, double-blind studies that compare synthetic levothyroxine to desiccated thyroid in terms of effectiveness at resolving patient symptoms. So despite orthodox claims to rely on science, the fact is that science doesn't exist to bolster the arguments that levothyroxine is clinically superior to desiccated thyroid.

But things have got worse: much worse. Today, the profession has such an obsession with blood tests and lab work—and such a total belief in their accuracy and supremacy, that it has become considered quackery to ignore them. A doctor who administers thyroid supplements to a patient, when the blood tests are "normal" faces censure and loss of the right to practice medicine.

To treat a patient properly with clinically severe hypothyroidism may be as much as a physician's license is worth. To diagnose by the signs of the disease (the only reliable diagnostic method) is a lost art and patients face having their symptoms put down to aging and inadequacy. Some patients are even taken off thyroid replacement therapy because they "don't need it any more"; the blood tests have "normalized".

So the poor patient's worthwhile life is ended, crucified on the cross of stupid and ignorant dogma. He or she piles on the weight, declines in energy, looks, vitality, joy and sexuality; cholesterol soars; a heart attack becomes almost inevitable.

Dose

I don't really feel I can recommend thyroid supplementation as a go-it-alone venture. You need skilled medical help. The trouble is, as I have indicated, that doctors are all but banned from helping struggling patients with thyroid issues.

But to guide you with dosing, if you can find a physician to sign off on it, read the following carefully...

It is always wise to start on a smaller dose of desiccated thyroid than they will ultimately need, such as 1 grain (60 mg). This will help the body get used to the supplement and there may be other issues which can reveal themselves, such as sluggish adrenals or low ferritin/iron levels.

But you will need to raise the dose quite soon, otherwise hypothyroid symptoms can return, due to the internal feedback loop in your body, which can happen if you stay on a low dose too long. Go to 2 grains in two or three weeks at most. Then 3 grains for a further four weeks, to give the needed variant T4 time to build (which can take 4-6 weeks). It's unlikely indeed that anyone would need more than 5 grains.

You can just swallow the grains or take them sublingually. When taking desiccated thyroid extract, it is important to avoid iron, estrogen and calcium supplements at the same time, since all bind the thyroid hormones to some degree.

You are looking for the removal of your hypothyroid symptoms, an afternoon temp of 98.6, a morning before-rising temp of 97.8 – 98.2 (depending on which method was used), good heart rate and blood pressure, good energy, clearing of brain fog, etc.

A good website for self-help information and notes is: www.stopthethyroidmadness.com, run by Janie Bowthorpe. She knows more than me! (She should, she suffered thyroid Hell herself and has made a career out of learning the full thyroid story).

Testosterone and "Male Estrogen"

The middle-aged paunch of men is well known. Male obesity has a different pattern to that of women; it lies to the front, whereas women fatten more at the side and hips. The male distribution is that of the classic "pot belly". It's part of the so-called andropause (male menopause).

There is no question that lifestyle factors play a part in male obesity: excess beer and pretzels, sedentary habits and so forth. But declining testosterone levels are also a key factor. This important male hormone is known to protect against obesity, as well as other dangers, such as hypertension and heart disease.

Men can become trapped in a vicious spiral of low testosterone leading to obesity; obesity further reduces testosterone levels (see below); and that leads to more obesity.

In spite of this widespread threat to men's health, most physicians do not test for testosterone levels in their obese male patients. If they did, millions of men could be protected against the scourge of metabolic syndrome (section 6), type 2 diabetes, high blood pressure, atherosclerosis, and cancer.

The popular medical myth has it that testosterone levels are directly associated with the death rate among men. Too much testosterone and you will die early is the perception. It's nonsense, through and through. According to one study, low testosterone is associated with almost 50% increase in mortality over a seven year period.[1]

Bottom line: low T is unquestionably associated with male obesity. So much so, that men over forty fighting obesity should get their testosterone levels checked and push their doctor towards supplementing any deficiency. But uneducated doctors fight shy of this, quoting absurd science such as testosterone replacement therapy "causes" testicular cancer.

This is nonsense and a myth hanging over from the days when testosterone replacement therapy was done by using the synthetic drug methyl testosterone. I don't want to go into the shabby ethics and false science behind drug companies altering safe natural molecules to make them patentable, solely for the pursuit of profits.

Suffice it to say that supplementation with unaltered natural testosterone, as for example using a cream or patch, is quite safe. Moreover there are several proven safe variations of the hormone, such as the proprionate, cyprionate and enanthate forms (usually by injection).

Note: This author deplores the use of testosterone supplement for anabolic enhancement (body building).

The "Male Estrogen" Problem

The story as described is destructive enough. But in fact things are even more complicated. One of the metabolites of testosterone—dihydrotestosterone or DHT—is a feminizing estrogen-type hormone. That's why older men start to develop breasts (man boobs) and lose their libido.

The drug that converts testosterone to the feminine form is called aromatase. It's not good; the less it does, the better. But obviously, if you take testosterone supplementally, there is a danger of even more DHT.

There are ways to protect against this. These range from drugs which inhibit aromatase, like Arimidex (anastrozole), to herbs and minerals. Zinc, for instance, helps keep aromatase in check. Unfortunately, more than 60 percent of men have a zinc deficiency. And that spells trouble... Your semen has 100 times more zinc than your blood – and your prostate has the highest concentration of zinc in your body.

A healthy level of zinc has the following benefits:

- Maximizes testosterone production
- Extends the life of testosterone in the bloodstream
- Boosts the sensitivity of male hormone receptors – especially your testosterone receptors[2]

You can also consider the following herbs as part of your program, the benefits of which have been well established in maintaining prostate health.

Chrysin (from the passion flower), which is well known to inhibit the enzyme aromatase.[3]

Bodybuilders have used chrysin as a testosterone-boosting supplement because, by inhibiting the aromatase enzyme, less testosterone is converted into estrogen.

Carnitine. Both testosterone and carnitine improve sexual desire, sexual satisfaction, and nocturnal penile tumescence, but carnitine is more effective than testosterone in improving erectile function, nocturnal penile tumescence, orgasm, and general sexual well-being. Carnitine was better than testosterone at treating depression.[4]

Skullcap (*Scutellaria baicalensis*) or Chinese skullcap. It has been shown to block the effect of the enzyme 5 alpha-reductase, another enzyme which acts like aromatase and converts testosterone to feminizing dihydrotestosterone.

Estrogen Dominance

Womens' hormonal problems are proverbial. Due to outrageous marketing lies, hammered home over many decades, women have been conditioned to believe that hormone replacements are the answer to almost all their misery. The least symptom and doctors will hastily prescribe estrogen in one form or another.

The story is so loaded with confusion and false information, that I think it's right to say most doctors don't understand this physiology properly. Their prescribing is way off-key.

While it is true that estrogen levels will decrease during menopause, estrogen levels do not fall significantly until after a woman's last period.

The real problem for most women is the opposite of this scenario: she has *too much estrogen*. At least too much in relation to available progesterone, a second hormone, which balances the bad effects of estrogen. The result is a condition we call "estrogen dominance", a term that was coined by John R. Lee MD, author of the now-famous book, *What Your Doctor May Not Tell You About Menopause*. It can start as early as age 35.

Symptoms Of Estrogen Dominance

Remember estrogen stimulates both brain and body, so psychological symptoms are common and often predominate; mood swings are among the commonest of all hormone-related symptoms in a woman but there can be fatigue, depression, loss of libido and brain fog.

What concerns us in this context is the sluggish metabolism, water retention, metabolic syndrome and weight gain (particularly around the abdomen and hips). These tend to go hand in hand with lowered thyroid function, creating a complex array of unpleasant and life-is-no-fun-any-more symptomatology.

As well as obesity, estrogen dominance has also been linked to allergies, autoimmune disorders, breast cancer, uterine cancer, infertility, ovarian cysts, and increased blood clotting, and accelerated aging.

Ironically, there is a vicious circle, because obesity is actually a cause of estrogen dominance, owing to its highly inflammatory nature, which I described earlier.

Progesterone Replacement

So you might think, from what I have said, that progesterone replacement is an easy way to go.

True! But be very, very careful. It all depends what you mean by progesterone. The natural hormone is very safe and can be found through all good holistic doctors and compounding pharmacies (local laws permitting).

But the waters are made incredibly muddy by the introduction of synthetic hormonal compounds called progestins. They have been indiscriminately used in birth control pills and HRT since the 1960s. Natural progesterone is just that: natural, meaning it can't be patented and sold for outrageous profits by pharmaceutical companies.

So they screw around with the chemistry and have formulated unnatural compounds, made from testosterone, which they can then patent and "own". These phony testosterone-derivative substances are called progestins. They are marketed falsely as "progesterone", ignorant doctors prescribe them, and women get sick.

Because, at the end of the day, these synthetic hormones, are not the real deal. They have some progesterone properties but not all. Worse than that: they are dogged with unpleasant side effects not found with the natural substance. Common problems include abdominal bloating, painful breasts, water retention, mood swings, fatigue, depression, rashes and dry skin, diarrhea, constipation, anxiety and pains in the joints and muscles.

Not good, I'm sure you will agree. But hardly surprising; progestins are not found anywhere in nature. The body does not respond well to them. Yet, that's all doctors prescribe because there are "proper" drugs (in the pharmacopeia).

It's worse still: progestins are in many ways more potent than natural progesterone and they actually inhibit the function of natural progesterone. So when the clumsy doctor steps in and prescribes these substances, nature is thwarted in her good intent. It means there is no use taking something like the birth control pill or HRT and expecting a natural progesterone supplement to work. It won't.

What Can You Do

It's important to bear in mind, if you are struggling with weight problems, that estrogen dominance may be an issue (even in men). To limit the scale of its impact, you must engage in certain health behaviors:

1. Limit your chemical exposure by filtering water, choosing only natural cosmetics where possible and using eco-friendly low-impact cleaning substances.

2. Supplement with natural progesterone, which is not something you should do without help from a competent health practitioner.

3. Aim to reduce your stress levels. It's been shown to increase the effect of estrogen dominance and inhibit the secretion of progesterone

4. Increase your intake of magnesium, B Vitamins, Zinc and Vitamin E as these all tend to be low in the presence of too much estrogen.

5. Exercise more, lowering body fat can help reduce the negative effects of estrogen.

6. Eat lots of "cruciferous" vegetables such as cabbage, Brussels sprouts, cauliflower, and broccoli. These vegetables may help to protect the body against estrogen and estrogen- dependent cancer because they contain diindolylmethane (DIM) and a related chemical called indole-3-carbinol. DIM promotes beneficial estrogen metabolism in both sexes by reducing the levels of 16-hydroxy estrogen metabolites (bad) and increasing the formation of 2-hydroxy estrogen metabolites (good), also resulting in increased antioxidant activity. That's according to the official government Cancer Institute website.[5]

Hormone Disruptors

As if all this isn't bad enough, we have an additional problem today: what are called hormone disruptors. You've probably heard the term; I'm referring to chemicals dumped in our environment which have a biological impact by mimicking our hormones or by interfering with their proper action.

Not all pesticides and pollutant chemicals may be threatening because they poison us; some get into our metabolic pathways and screw up normal healthy functions, including the action of our hormones.

The knowledgeable scientists today will accept that data shows conclusively that the current epidemic in obesity cannot be explained solely by alterations in food intake and/or decrease in exercise. Nor can it be just a genetic question. True, there is a genetic predisposition component of obesity; but genetics could not have altered so dramatically over just the past few decades. On the other hand, environmental changes—from the rise of modern food packaging, to what I have christened the "chemical blizzard" which we are all subjected to—might be responsible for at least part of the current obesity epidemic.

It's a smoking gun!

Chemicals are noted that appear to cause weight gain by interfering with elements of the human weight control system—such as alterations in weight-balancing hormones, altered sensitivity to neurotransmitters, or altered activity of the sympathetic nervous system.

For example, certain substances free in the environment today, act like estrogens (so-called xenoestrogens). We've already seen earlier in this section the problems that estrogen dominance can bring about, including fluid retention and weight gain. So that last thing we need is more estrogens, especially when their origin is disguised and hidden.

But it's worse yet: environmental pollutants, including estrogen mimics, affect everybody; that means males and females alike, sexually undeveloped and sexually mature alike. Think this through: males are getting pumped with estrogen too; not good. Children (before puberty) are getting flooded with estrogens; definitely not good.

Even babies in the womb are getting hit with unnatural estrogens. So much so, that proper anatomical development is being perverted. Infant boys are being born with mis-formed genitals at an unprecedented rate; it's as if male infants are trying to change their mind and be born as females instead. The testes are poorly formed and the penis may be missing altogether.

These malformations have always occurred, but not at the alarming rate we see them today. Any intelligent, thinking scientist is under no illusions: estrogen pollution of the environment is the cause of this distressing rise in these semi-males.

Such pollution compounds include well-known BPA (bisphenol A), phthalates and PCBs (polychlorinated hydroxybiphenyls). Until the halt of their US manufacture in 1977, PCBs were commonly used as lubricants and coolants in a wide variety of electrical equipment including common household items. Due to a very long half-life PCBs were found to build up in the environment, specifically in soil, sediment, and water, where they still exist today.

Xenoestrogens are also found in household products, or their breakdown derivatives, such as nonylphenol and octylphenol.

You need to get these out of your life and that means drinking only glass-bottled waters and filtering your tapwater cleanly. Do not use plastic bottled spring waters as a substitute, because of their phthalate content.

Don't forget that xenoestrogens, or foreign estrogens, are also found in plant foodstuffs: they are called phytoestrogens and occur naturally in plants such as clover, soybeans and other legumes, whole grains and many fruits and vegetables.

Recycled Hormones

It's a little-known fact that toilet effluent (sewage) contains the residues of most drugs, including replacement hormones. Since hormones are very powerful and create their effect with just trace amounts, this becomes a significant extra hormone burden. It's a bad joke that even men take the contraceptive pill daily, due to what is flushed down the toilet and re-appears in tapwater!

You must get an adequate water cleansing system, preferably using reverse osmosis (RO), plus an activated charcoal filter.

Water filtration jugs are barely adequate and, although they are sold honestly and ethically, cannot properly cope with today's tide of pollutants in our drinking water systems.

Water Filtration

That leaves us to clean up our own water: water filtration.

The simplest kind to use is a filtration jug, such as the German Brita® water filter. These models use an activated carbon filter, which is good for taking out chemicals, but not very efficient. Really, jug filters are only designed to make your water taste better. They do filter to a degree but cannot **purify** water passed through them.

The same is true of fridge filters.

And, of course, the performance of these simple filters falls off with time. As the filter accumulates toxic waste, they are less and less efficient, like a car oil filter collecting dirt.

A better grade of filtration is RO or reverse osmosis. My good friend Robert Slovak is the Daddy of RO filter science. He and his late brother Jack have watched the industry grow, until we now have state-of-the-art water filtration, using a combination of activated carbon and an RO set-up.

What does reverse osmosis mean? Briefly (and not too technically) it means water forced through a special membrane, which is designed to separate it from all chemical contaminants, right down to the molecular level. So it's not just for removing solids but chemicals too. And it can do this very efficiently.

Truly, RO filtration is the standard we want to go to. The best I know is the model called the AquaTru®:

The AquaTru® outperforms practically any other filtration system you can name. With the size and convenience of a counter-top unit (only slightly larger than the biggest Brita system) the days of filter jugs are over. RO is the standard!

The AquaTru® is not slow: it can filter 2 quarts of water in just 15 minutes. That's a huge leap forwards on other RO systems.

Learn more about the AquaTru® here: https://www.alternative-doctor.com/bestwater/

PART 2. THE ISSUES

SECTION 12. HOW YOUR GUT FLORA MAY MAKE YOU FAT

I promised you some staggering new science that could throw open the whole debate on the origins of obesity and this one factor could be the most important breakthrough discovery of all, paving the way to simple, easy and controlled weight loss.

Are you ready for this?

Altered bowel flora due to the abuse and overuse of antibiotics.

Why would taking penicillin, sulfa drugs, cephalosporins, streptomycin and all the brouhaha of modern antimicrobials lead to obesity? Ah, that's an interesting and surprising story.

What's more, it's not just a story of medical blunders—overprescribing and abuse by doctors. Did you know that over 75% of antibiotics that are manufactured go to agricultural uses? What's more, they are fed to animals that are otherwise entirely healthy. Why?

Profits, of course. Animals fed small traces of antibiotics grow up heavier and fatter than untreated animals. Yes, I know what you are thinking... if taking routine antibiotics fattens up commercial livestock, won't it fatten up humans too?

Dead right. And that's what has been happening. Trouble is, for both animals and humans, taking antibiotics wipes out huge colonies of healthy microbes that we need, living in our intestines. They may be creepy and slimy, but they belong there and are important for our health; the same way that earthworms, even though they slither around and are "Eeeuw!" to pick up, are vital for the healthy condition of the soils in which we grow our crops.

This is an example of where "Yucky" is good!

These important microbes help us keep in balance with our diet; some of them even help by digesting our food, making available key nutrients, like vitamin K, and helping us steer the path away from weight gain.

To find out more about this, let's dive into the next section...

The Good Guys and The Bad Guys

It has been found that we harbor several strains of bacteria in our gut. Two strains are especially important in this context: the so-called *Bacteriodes* and the *Firmicutes*.

Briefly, individuals with lots of *Firmicutes* strains gain weight far too easily; those with mostly *Bacteroides* are much better off and won't gain weight, even on the same diet. So you will see right away that extensive use of antibiotics carries the hazard of damaging and changing the balance of gut flora in unfavorable ways. Antibiotics can trigger weight problems... Hello! Another hidden pathway (at least nobody seems to be properly seeing it, till now) which might explain our current obesity epidemic! Antibiotics which kill mostly *Firmicutes* would result in weight gain, even eating exactly the same diet as before.

The thing is, bacteria in the intestine play a crucial role in digestion. They provide enzymes necessary for the uptake of many nutrients, synthesize certain vitamins and boost absorption of energy from food. Fifty years ago, farmers learned that by tweaking the microbial mix in their livestock with low-dose oral antibiotics, they could accelerate weight gain. So the fact that we are encountering low-level antibiotics in our food and water supplies is very bad news from the point of view of unwanted weight gain.

Maybe we are just like cattle and tending to gain weight because of constant exposure to antibiotics?

In a 2012 study, published in the journal *Nature Immunology*, a research team based at the University of Chicago was able to unravel some of the mechanisms that regulate this type of weight gain. They focused on the relationship between the immune system, gut bacteria, digestion and obesity. They showed how weight gain requires not just caloric overload but also a delicate, adjustable and transmissible, interplay between intestinal microbes and the immune response. [1]

Obesity Is a Type of Infection

So, is there a connection between the last 60 years of excessive antibiotic use (abuse) and the current obesity epidemic? Seems the answer is a resounding YES.

You can become "infected" with weight gain! If you harbor weight-gain microbes in your gut, you will have a problem. The thing is, it's not really an infection mechanism but an inflammation mechanism; let me explain.

A team of researchers at Emory, Cornell University and the University of Colorado at Boulder, led by Andrew Gewirtz, became intrigued by the relationship between gut bugs and weight when they noticed that lab mice with a certain level of inflammation in their bodies had more bugs than other animals and were about 15% heavier. Inflammatory signaling can promote metabolic syndrome, which you have learned about in these pages, and which causes weight gain, high blood pressure and high cholesterol levels and a higher risk for developing diabetes and heart disease.

In a way, inflammatory factors and insulin compete for the attention of the same intestinal cells; if the cells are busy responding to inflammatory factors, then they are less likely to take up glucose and process it effectively.

It's not that the bacteria are directly making the mice eat more but that the bacteria are causing low-grade inflammation, which causes insulin resistance and that makes the mice eat more.

What was even more convincing was that, when the gut flora of the fat mice was transplanted to healthy normal-weight mice, they too became fat! So you really can "catch" obesity. It's just that inflammation seems to be the underlying mechanism. [2]

Don't run away with the idea that it's just antibiotics that do the damage, though they are a major factor, unquestionably. It's also the immune system, that is supposed to fight rampant bacterial populations, that may be at fault.

And that explains why my own diet plan (section 5)—avoiding allergy foods or inflammatory foods—often brings immediate weight loss benefits. The immune system is nurtured by unburdening it from lots of bad foods. It bounces back, gets a hold of the situation and bowel flora comes under control once more.

Plus, it lessens inflammation, by removing foods that cause allergic reactions. Makes a lot of sense.

Fiber, The Microbiome and Weight Loss

I remember an English comedian (Jasper Carrot) talking about Audrey Eyton's "F-Plan Diet", back in the 1980s. We need to eat more fiber, she told us. Beans for breakfast, beans for lunch, beans for supper, beans with everything... No wonder it's called the F-Plan, he laughed! (farting, get it?)

I used to joke differently, that if fiber was all it took, we'd just need to chop up the carpets and eat those and we'd all be healthy. I thought there must be more to it than that... And so there is.

If you are confused by it all, you won't be after reading this. Dietary fiber has been a much misunderstood nutrient. Many people know it is important, but not much more than that. It's time to straighten it all out and make it nice and simple.

Fiber digestion is crucial to our gut microbiome.

What Is Fiber?

Dietary fiber, also known as roughage or bulk, includes all parts of plant foods that your body can't digest or absorb. Unlike other food components, such as fats, proteins or carbohydrates, fiber isn't digested by your body. Instead, it passes relatively intact through your stomach, small intestine, colon and out of the other end.

That's the whole point. Fiber helps to maintain a solid formed stool, instead of just spludge from your back passage or— even worse—concreted, hard rocks that you can pass only with extreme difficulty.

So it's a part of the process of stool formation but not involved in the carbs, proteins and fats digestion story. Actually, my joke about eating carpets comes close to how you need to picture this.

So what? You might ask. Well, actually fiber is important in many ways, we have discovered over the years. It helps with weight loss, lowers cholesterol, prevents heart disease, lessens the risk of cancer and diabetes, improves digestion and greatly benefits our gut flora, for a start.

Pay attention, this is important!

Soluble vs. Insoluble Fiber

There are two main types of fiber: soluble and insoluble. Soluble fiber dissolves in water; insoluble fiber does not. Both are beneficial for health but each in different ways.

Soluble fiber attracts water and forms a gel, which slows down digestion. Soluble fiber delays the emptying of your stomach and makes you feel full, which helps control weight. Slower stomach emptying may also affect blood sugar levels and have a beneficial effect on insulin sensitivity, which may help control diabetes. Soluble fibers can also help lower LDL ("bad") blood cholesterol.

Sources of soluble fiber include: oatmeal, oat cereal, lentils, apples, oranges, pears, oat bran, strawberries, nuts, flaxseeds, beans, dried peas, blueberries, psyllium husk, cucumbers, celery, and carrots.

Insoluble fibers are considered gut-healthy fiber because they have a laxative effect and add bulk to the diet, helping prevent constipation. These fibers do not dissolve in water, so they pass through the gastrointestinal tract relatively intact, and speed up the passage of food and waste through your gut. Insoluble fibers are mainly found in whole grains and vegetables.

Sources of insoluble fiber include: whole wheat, whole grains, wheat bran, corn bran, seeds, nuts, barley, couscous, brown rice, bulgur, zucchini, celery, broccoli, cabbage, onions, tomatoes, carrots, cucumbers, green beans, dark leafy vegetables, raisins, grapes, fruit, and root vegetable skins.

Some plants contain significant amounts of both soluble and insoluble fiber. For example plums and prunes have insoluble fiber in the skin and soluble fiber in the pulp.

Synthetic Fiber Products

You probably know about psyllium husks, loved by doctors because it is a "real" drug and prescribable! They like Inulin too, because it's "real" (see below).

There are some other odd products on the market, such as glucomannan, an extract of the konjac plant (also known as konjaku, konnyaku, or the konnyaku potato). It is a water-soluble mixture of glucose and mannose and is considered a fiber product.

Japanese shirataki noodles (also marketed as "miracle noodles") are made from glucomannan. You can put these gooey noodles with anything and assume them to be zero calories. They lack flavor though.

In one 2007 study of glucomannan, published in the *British Journal of Nutrition,* participants taking a glucomannan and psyllium husk combination supplement lost approximately 10 pounds in 16 weeks compared to 1.7 pounds lost in the placebo group. [3]

Another study using only glucomannan showed an average of 5.5 pounds lost over eight weeks, without making any other diet or lifestyle changes. [4]

Vegetable gum fiber supplements are also relatively new to the market. Often sold as a powder, vegetable gum fibers dissolve easily with no aftertaste. In preliminary clinical trials, they have proven effective for the treatment of irritable bowel syndrome. [5]

How Much?

We need about 30 – 40 grams of fiber a day; women somewhat less than men and we all need less as we grow older. Most Westerners get 20 grams or less: not enough.

But don't suddenly up your intake, otherwise you will be blowing off (breaking wind) and upsetting those around you. Increase your intake slowly towards the optimum and take plenty of water at the same time; soluble fiber needs that and despite what you have read, it isn't easy to pass soluble fiber, if water is short. It will swell and tend to block the intestine, which is the opposite of what is wanted.

As I said, most plants contain both soluble and insoluble fiber. However, the amount of each type varies in different plant foods. If you focus on eating a healthy diet rich in fruits, vegetables, whole grains, legumes, nuts, and seeds, you will certainly take in plenty of fiber.

Remember, animals, fowl and fish contain no worthwhile fiber.

Weight Loss Benefits

One of the great things about eating fiber is it gives that pleasant full feeling, without actually adding to your calories. High-fiber foods generally require more chewing, which gives your body time to register when you're no longer hungry, so you're less likely to overeat.

In conjunction with leaving you feeling more satisfied, fiber helps properly regulate our weight-control hormones, such as insulin, ghrelin and leptin. Fiber foods can slow the absorption of sugar and help improve blood sugar levels. So a healthy diet that includes fiber may reduce the risk of developing type 2 diabetes.

Slimmer's need to understand the importance of fiber foods and choose carefully from among them. Fruits and veggies enjoy no great reputation but plant foods are essential for the fiber ingredient they bring.

Pre-Biotics vs. Probiotic

Now we come to the real reason that fiber is important to health. I believe this part of the story is much more relevant than just the idea of chopped up carpets! Fiber is a pre-biotic.

Definition: a pre-biotic is a non-digestible food ingredient that stimulates the healthy growth and/ or activity of bacteria in the digestive system in ways beneficial to overall health. The term (and concept) was coined by Marcel Roberfroid in 1995. [6]

A probiotic, on the other hand, is defined as a valuable microorganism that lives in the gut symbiotically, that is sharing our digestive milieu without parasitic stealing.

Factually, most pre-biotics belong to the biochemical class of oligosaccharides (short-chain carbohydrates, mostly indigestible).

The pre-biotic definition does not emphasize a specific bacterial group. Generally, however, it is assumed that a pre-biotic should increase the number and/or activity of bifidobacteria and lactic acid bacteria. The importance of the bifidobacteria and the lactic acid bacteria (LABs) is that these groups of bacteria may have several beneficial effects on the host, especially in terms of improving digestion, including enhancing mineral absorption [7] and the effectiveness and intrinsic strength of the immune system.[8]

Both types of fiber benefit healthy bowel flora but more so the soluble type.

Traditional dietary sources of pre-biotics include soybeans, inulin sources (such as Jerusalem artichoke, jicama, and chicory root), raw oats, unrefined (whole) wheat, unrefined barley, and yacon.

It is interesting to note that the ONLY non-plant source of suitable pre-biotic oligosaccharides is human breast milk and these are believed to play an important role in the development of a healthy immune system in infants. [9]

Finally, Best Probiotics And Where To Get 'Em

You'll read lots of claims for probiotic substances; just be wary of what you buy.

Ilya Metchnikoff, a Russian immunologist, started all this, with his theories about yoghurt and the bacterium *Lactobacillus acidophilus*. He claimed that Bulgarians lived long and stayed healthy due to their consumption of a particular Lactobacillus strain he named *L. bulgaricus*, a highly doubtful conclusion from the epidemiological evidence available to him.

Zaro Agha, a Turk, was once believed to be the oldest person in modern times. According to *Time Magazine* (March 17, 1930), having reached the age of 162. He attributed his longevity to eating massive amounts of yogurt all his life!

Agha was born two years before the signing of the American Declaration of Independence, and lived until 1934. He stayed physically active, working as a porter in Istanbul, a physically demanding job which he held for 100 years. Zaro was the subject of much scientific and popular curiosity.

Metchnikoff established a relationship between disease and harmful bacteria in the bowel, and postulated that friendly probiotic bacteria which are in yogurt can neutralize the disease-causing bacteria and thus prolong the normal lifespan.

Metchnikoff shared the 1908 Nobel Prize for Physiology and Medicine with Paul Ehrlich for his breakthroughs in understanding the human immune system. Metchnikoff was decades ahead of his time.

Only today are we really seeing the emergence of scientific support for the fact that our bowel bacteria, or "intestinal flora" as it's called, is probably the number one issue in health. Good bowel flora: good health and longevity; bad bowel flora: disease, inflammation and an early death. It's that simple.

Today, yoghurt continues to enjoy a good reputation for promoting health. It's widely assumed that it acts as a probiotic; that is, it provides healthy safe bowel commensal organisms, which help squeeze out any unwanted nasty microbes in our gut space.

Yakult

Enter Dr. Minoru Shirota (1899-1982), working in a microbiology lab at Kyoto Imperial University's School of Medicine in Japan. He became the first in the world to succeed in culturing a particular strain of lactic acid bacteria beneficial to human health, which he called "Lactobacillus casei, strain Shirota" or LcS.

His discovery led to the development of Yakult, an affordable mass-market fermented milk drink, which was introduced to the market in 1935. It is still on sale today.

It has some science too. Searching PubMed, the medical online database, returned over 100 studies of LcS, like this one:

"To evaluate the effect of probiotics on the prevention of carcinogenesis, Lactobacillus casei Shirota (LcS) was given to the patients who had undergone the resection of superficial bladder cancer, and administration of LcS significantly reduced the recurrence rate of bladder cancer.

Daily ingestion of fermented milk containing LcS restored NK cell activity (natural killer cells, needed for the fight against cancer). The researchers stated, "These findings suggest that LcS may help the reinforcement of our defense system against cancer by modulating innate immune functions."[10]

Modern Paragons

Today, we would look to *Lactobacillus rhamnosus 35* (Mcr35), made in Aurillac in France, as the Rolls-Royce of probiotics, or to BB12 (Bifidobacterium lactis 12). Bif makes sense, rather than lactobacillus, because about 90% of our natural flora is Bif. Human-friendly probiotics are better tolerated and survive well in our gut, whereas cow's milk derived organisms, typical of most yoghurts and so-called probiotics, don't last. Sorry Metchnikoff!

So Can Probiotics Help Weight Loss?

Yes. A team of Japanese researchers split 210 overweight people into three groups. While everyone consumed a daily 7-ounce serving of fermented milk, two of the groups drank milk spiked with varying amounts of a probiotic called *Lactobacillus gasseri SBT2055*, which past research has tied to fat loss. After 12 weeks, people taking the probiotic milk formulas dropped roughly 8 to 9 percent of their visceral fat. Both probiotic groups also lost 1 to 3 percent of their belly fat, the study shows.

How does it do that? It's possible the probiotic featured in the study lowers intestinal inflammation and aids digestion, both of which could prevent the buildup of body fat.

Unfortunately, the probiotic strain highlighted in this research isn't commercially available in the U.S. right now.

Also note, there are some contradictory studies. A paper published in 2011 in the *International Journal of Obesity* found that while some strains of probiotics aid weight loss, others contribute to obesity. "The research now is premature, and requires more analysis," says that study's co-author, Didier Raoult, MD, PhD, a Marseille, France- based microbiologist.[11]

Thing is: probiotics offer benefits to be sure. But the jury's still out on how much probiotics help when it comes to weight loss. There is definitely a role for probiotics in dieting. But scientists are still teasing apart all the mechanisms involved. So for now, don't count on a probiotic to replace your treadmill or diet plan.

Hey! One other reason probiotics may help you lose weight...

Probiotics Calm Your Thoughts!

A study from UCLA, published in the journal *Gastroenterology*, researchers divided 36 healthy women between the ages of 18 and 55 into three groups. One group ate yogurt containing a mix of several probiotics twice a day for four weeks, another consumed a dairy product that looked and tasted like yogurt but contained no probiotics, and the third group had no yogurt products.

At the end of the four weeks, the women's brains were scanned and when the researchers compared the scans with ones taken before the trial, they found that those who had eaten the yogurt with probiotics had a decrease in activity in the area of the brain that controls emotion, cognition, and sensory feelings in response to the emotion-recognition test. Those who had no probiotics had an increase in activity, meaning they had more negative emotional reactions.

Yoghurt (probiotics) were clearly rewarding emotionally and probably help against stress and anxiety: two of the main reasons for comfort eating! So maybe it would be smart to introduce probiotics anyway. But there's a caution; you need to read and understand my section on food allergy (major cause of weight gain), where you will learn allergies to milk and dairy products is widespread.

So maybe hold off till you know whether you tolerate dairy or not.

Coconut Oil To The Rescue

A new study from the University of Belgrade in the Republic of Serbia, published in the journal *Plant Foods for Human Nutrition* on August 31, 2018, with the title Beneficial Effect of Virgin Coconut Oil on Alloxan-Induced Diabetes and Microbiota Composition in Rats adds further proof, if it were needed, that virgin coconut oil is a powerful remedy for diabetes and helps control obesity. [12]

In this latest study, virgin coconut oil was shown to be beneficial to the microbiome by increasing probiotic bacteria, leading to better outcomes for those suffering with diabetes.

This new research confirms what many have reported to us over the past 15 plus years, that virgin coconut oil is beneficial in overcoming both Type 1 and Type 2 diabetes.

This new study offers a possible explanation as to how virgin coconut oil helps people with Type 1 diabetes without directly affecting insulin levels.

Interestingly, the coconut oil didn't do much for the blood sugar levels. But the microbiome was very positively affected, significantly increased the abundance of probiotic bacteria, such as Lactobacillus, Allobaculum, and Bifidobacterium species.

Another study (Dec 2017, same journal) showed the amazing benefits of coconut oil against metabolic syndrome, using rats. Virgin coconut oil was found to lower body weight, blood glucose concentrations and systolic blood pressure, with improved structure and function of the heart and liver.[13]

Despite mainstream naysayers, the importance of intestinal microbiome composition in the treatment of type 2 diabetes has been undeniably emphasized.

Understanding The Context

Type 2 diabetes is the result of poor lifestyle and dietary habits that lead to metabolic syndrome or insulin resistance syndrome, and then type 2 diabetes. The problem is not with insufficient insulin, like in Type 1 diabetes; there is no drop off in pancreatic production of insulin.

In other words, type 2 diabetics have enough insulin, and sometimes more than enough (hyperinsulinemia). But the cells that need to metabolize glucose with oxygen and produce energy aren't able to pack-in the insulin that is supposed to escort glucose molecules into the cells.

The results could be via the inflammation mechanism (type 1 diabetes is highly inflammatory in nature). Animal studies show clearly that coconut oil is protective against systemic inflammation (section 7), even if it's added to an unhealthy diet of convenience, such as the standard American diet or SAD.

Of course this is not to advocate the "recklessly poor" SAD diet. It serves as a scientific observation that eliminating processed carbohydrates and high fructose corn syrup while using coconut oil should create a strong foundation for better health and immunity from one's diet. Plus weight loss is almost guaranteed.

Quick and Simple Diet #4. Give Up Alcohol

Many a man has found that just coming off the booze for a few weeks results in the pounds tumbling off. No question: too much beer is fattening. Moreover, it plays dirty tricks with your hormones and metabolism (low-T, for example). And it impairs function, of course. Shakespeare had the night porter in the play *Macbeth* (act 2, scene 3) famously remark: "It provokes the desire, but it takes away the performance" (makes you horny but results in you being a poor lover).

It's not just beer; cocktails too can be loaded with unwanted calories and carbs. The average serving of spirits (vodka, rum, gin, etc.) contains about 115 calories, even before the mixers have been added. Some cocktails contain more calories than a Big Mac. So ladies, beware: cocktails can add up to 500 calories or more (TGI Friday's "Ultimate Mudslide" clocks in at a massive 740 calories, while a Long Island Iced Tea tops even that, at 789 cals.)[14]

A better bet, if you want to drink, is good wines and champagne. Everyone knows about the "French paradox", the fact that the French are (or used to be) slim on the whole, yet eat well and drink large quantities of wine, per capita. A standard 6 oz. (175 mls.) glass of wine is around 150 calories but can be as high as 300 calories, depending on the wine.

Set this against the fact that a beer comes in at around 100 calories per 12 oz pour. You'll have to search the internet for listings, to find the exact score of your favorite tipple.

All of which is unimportant, if you decide to avoid alcohol as a weight-loss strategy. And it is certainly a "quick and simple" approach. Remember, a gram of alcohol has 7 calories, while a gram of carbohydrates or protein each has only 4 calories; fat has 9 calories; not much more than alcohol!

What this boils down to is that if you drink around 2 – 3 units a day, you'll lose weight immediately, just by quitting.

What to drink? Well, avoid switching to fruit juices; those are basically sugar drinks. There are only three meaningful alternatives (cheap and easy to obtain): tea, coffee and water. Tea should be black, or if you are not sure you can stomach that, try herbal infusions, such as peppermint, chamomile or Tulsi (holy basil).

Coffee is also best drunk black. But you can also avoid dairy (milk) by using soya milk, almond milk or one of the other modern dairy substitutes. AT ALL COSTS YOU MUST AVOID FLAVORED SYRUPS IN COFFEE. "Pumpkin spiced latte", "Hazelnut" and all similar variants are loaded with unwanted calories and carbs. The syrup is usually high-fructose corn syrup (HFCS), that last thing a determined slimmer wants. It will also badly damage your liver.

Safest of all is water, sparkling or still. Poured from a glass bottle (like San Pellegrino, for example) is much preferred over drinking water from plastic bottles. You have already learned in section 7 about "obesogens" or "hormone disruptors" from plastics, which cause estrogenic effects (weight gain and water retention).

Filtered water is a specialized subject on its own: ideally you need reverse-osmosis water, finished with an activated carbon filter. On no account buy into the idea that distilled water is "pure" and therefore the best. We get quite a lot of minerals from our drinking water and some of these are essential for health. Distilled water removes everything, even the good stuff!

Here are some good reasons to drink water, apart from its zero calories:

It can help by creating the feeling of a full stomach, so you will eat less.

It helps balance body fluids, for optimum health.

Water keeps skin hydrated and glowing. Healthy skin needs plenty of water to keep the layers plump and looking good. Drinking more will prevent avoidable dryness and some wrinkles (cosmetic hydrating creams do not do this, despite the hype).

Finally, you need a plentiful supply of fluid to support your most vital detox organs—the kidneys. How much do you need? Enough that your urine is not yellow but pale and watery. Drink more if you have to.

PART 2. THE ISSUES

SECTION 13.
A FEW ORPHAN FACTORS IN OBESITY

Poor Sleep Makes You Fat!

Get plenty of sound sleep (but not too much) is the mantra. A faulty sleep pattern (too much or too little), we now know, will play a role in obesity and is in itself pro-inflammatory. A study published in the journal *Sleep* tracked adults' visceral fat over five years. People who slept five hours or less, or eight or more hours, per night gained more visceral fat than those who slept between six and seven hours per night.

Sleep deprivation has been found to induce, among other things:

An increase in levels of inflammation in the body. Inflammation in the body may participate in the poor functioning of hormones such as insulin resistance and leptin resistance, both of which as you have learned are implicated in obesity.[1]

In one study, just one night of about 4 hours sleep was enough to significantly impair insulin functioning. So this is serious.[2]

Lack of sleep causes raised levels of the "hungry" hormone ghrelin. [3] It lowers levels of the "I feel full" hormone leptin (an appetite-suppressing and metabolism- boosting hormone). [4]

In another study, stopping men sleeping for a single night led to them eating significantly more the following day. [5]

Sleep deprivation leads to increased levels of the stress hormone cortisol. Excess cortisol can cause deposition of belly fat.[6]

It also slows down the metabolism (burning up) of fats. In one study, reducing useful sleep time from 8 hours to 6½ hours caused the metabolism of fat to fall by two-thirds.[7]

As some researchers have suggested, changing sleep patterns over recent decades might be an important but under-recognized factor in the rising rates of obesity and chronic disease. [8]

Sleep Deprivation Leads To Unhealthy Shopping!

This sleep thing can be very subtle. A study from Sweden found that lack of sleep even led to unhealthy shopping choices! [9]

Fourteen men were given about $50 to spend on food in two different occasions: once after the men had a full night's sleep, and once after a night of complete sleep deprivation.

On each occasion, men were given a set breakfast in the morning, so that hunger would not be a factor in their choices. The study subjects were asked to purchase as much food as they could with the money they had available.

The results showed that after the night with insufficient sleep, the men purchased food that had a higher calorie content; 9% more, which might not sound much but it is enough to cause relentless weight gain, if that's more than you need.

To dig deeper, the researchers also measured morning levels of the appetite-stimulating hormone ghrelin (page 54). This was higher in the morning, overall, after the night without sleep. However, ghrelin levels did not correlate with purchasing decisions, so the higher levels of hormones doesn't really explain the effect of sleep deprivation on the poor choice of foods.

What Can You Do? (Tricks To Get More Sleep)

If you are struggling with weight issues and don't sleep too well, you must work on that. It's not a "waste of time" to have more sleep but rather a sensible investment in health and longevity. You might give up hundreds of hours now but you could get back years or even decades of healthy life. What a deal!

To ignore this burgeoning science about the effects of sleep deprivation on obesity would be rather foolish. Certainly it will make your weight loss efforts less effective or even doom them to failure.

What about bringing your habitual bedtime forward by an hour? I'm not talking about never having a late night. I'm talking about creating a new core lifestyle shift that will help with your weight problems.

Remember, also, there is emerging science making it clear that adequate sleep will ensure you live longer than those who suffer from insomnia. Plenty of reasons to get more shut-eye!

Binaural beats and other electronic devices to take you down to theta and then delta are also valuable tools. You can read more about these devices here:

http://www.alternative-doctor.com/getthekasina/

One step further would be to consider a sleep remedy. I'm not thinking of the ghastly (and dangerous) pharmaceutical drugs, like Ambien. But there are good formulas, such as Alteril: a mixture of melatonin, l-tryptophan and valerian root.

Magnesium can be a good sleep remedy too, don't forget: 400 mg an hour before bedtime could work wonders!

One of the best remedies I know, and one I use myself, is L-Theanine, an amino acid. It has no sedative action but it does induce theta brainwaves, the kind that appear just before falling asleep. It makes "dropping off" simple and natural (L-Theanine is found in tea, which could explain its calming effect!)

Take 100 or 200 mg L-Theanine at night (experiment which works best).

Sleep Apnea

Obstructive sleep apnea (OSA) is believed to also raise inflammatory levels, probably acting via visceral fat and adipokines. [10]

It may be a two-way traffic, in which sleep apnea causes weight gain but weight gain is a known predisposition factor for sleep apnea!

OSA is easily and beneficially corrected with dental adjustments or a constant positive airway pressure (CPAP) device. It can result in a small but significant decrease in obesity, BMI and abdominal fat. [11]

Can Parasites Cause Weight Gain?

Actually, they can. That might seem counterintuitive because you might be thinking in terms of parasites robbing the host of nutrients and the host therefore becoming emaciated and starved.

That happens too.

But parasites are tricky in many ways; they hide, they cheat, they rob and double-cross. So generally speaking, they are in the frame for any adverse human condition, either causing it or making it worse.

Parasites are often implicated in obesity problems. Many overweight persons infested with parasites are constantly hungry, which leads to overeating (because of the parasites).

Two things will clinch your understanding of this:

1. People who take vigorous steps to eliminate parasites will often shed many pounds as a result

2. Although parasites compete for your food, they take the best, leaving you with the residual equivalent of junk food.

So it's always a great idea to consider a parasite cleanse.

Where would you get parasites from? That's an easy answer. Parasites are found in commercial pork products (bacon, ham, hot dogs, cold cuts, pork chops, etc.), beef, chicken, lamb, and even fish are contaminated. Plus you can get infected from fresh vegetables and salads, through contaminated water. And if that's not enough, infected workers handling food and food products can contaminate your nutrient supplies.

Plus you can become infected from your pets: birds, cats and dogs...

Other Symptoms That May Suggest Parasites

Frequent diarrhea, chronic constipation, gas & bloating, abdominal pain, nausea, mucus in the stool, low energy, weakness, mental confusion, dry skin and hair, brittle hair and hair loss, muscle pain, joint pain, muscle cramps... the list, frankly, could go on and on and on. In a sense, they are just symptoms of a body experiencing overload.

Most striking, when seen, are the psychological symptoms that can be caused by parasites; depression, anxiety, confusion and sexual disorders. Protozoa, worms of all kinds, fungi and flukes can invade the brain and cause headaches and strange, unpleasant feelings, which doctors may then have trouble diagnosing, because they rarely think of parasites.

The best position to take is to assume at least the possibility of parasites and ask for help. Your doctor can easily fix up a lab test. Trouble is, many of these tests are carried out by hospital labs that are, well frankly, poor at detecting signs of parasites.

Conventional treatment is also a bit suspect. Most of it is effective, if taken in a sufficient dose, but then toxicity problems can arise at higher doses. What is poisonous to a worm is also likely to be poisonous to you!

It would be safer to consider a herbal formula. These have been around for centuries and have a proven track record. Just remember they too can be toxic.

Plus there is the problem of feeling bad due to killing large numbers of parasites all at once in your body. These mass deaths release a lot of toxins and you can end up feeling really bad due to that and maybe blame "the cure".

Here's An Irony To Finish

Some people in Hong Kong seek to deliberately infect themselves with parasites, in order to lose weight, the U.K.'s *Daily Telegraph* reported. Let me warn you against going to such extremes, even if you could face up to the idea. The consequences can be fatal.

The Hong Kong Department of Health said Chinese Web sites have been offering weight-loss products containing dangerous parasites as a way of shedding extra pounds. That's 180 degrees round from what I have been saying. Don't be confused; this is the loony fringe and greedy marketers in on the act.

The products on offer contain the eggs of Ascaris worms, giant intestinal roundworms, which can grow up to 15-inches inside a host's intestines and lay up to 200,000 eggs a day inside the body.

The unpleasant side effects of abdominal pain and distension, vomiting, diarrhea and malnutrition are the least you would want to worry about. Ascaris infestation may also be fatal if serious complications such as intestinal, biliary tract or pancreatic duct obstruction arise. The worms travel round the body and may even invade such remote organs as the lungs.

Don't do it!

Brown Adipose Tissue

Time to visit the brown fat story (brown adipose tissue).

One of the exciting research trends of this millennium has been finding the special properties of brown adipose tissue (BAT), or just brown fat. It is one of two types of fat that humans and other mammals have. Its main function is to turn food into body heat. It is sometimes called "good" fat.

In fact BAT has been recognized since 1551, when Swiss researcher Konrad Gessner first found its presence in hibernating animals. There was a frenzy of interest in the 1980s, which faded when it was supposed that BAT did not persist beyond childhood.

Now it's back, center stage.

White adipocytes, or white fat cells, have a single lipid droplet, but brown adipocytes contain many small lipid droplets, and a high number of iron-containing mitochondria. It is this high iron content that gives brown fat its dark red to tan color.

Brown fat has more capillaries than white fat, because of its higher oxygen consumption. Brown fat also has many unmyelinated nerves, providing autonomic (sympathetic) stimulation to the fat cells.

The fat that builds up around a person's waist and thighs is the white type. Brown fat mainly accumulates around the neck and shoulders.

The functions of brown fat have only recently started to become clear. The main differences between the two types of fat appear to be as follows:

1. White adipose tissue (WAT), or white fat is the result of storing excess calories. When we consume too many calories, the body converts them into an energy reserve in the form of white fat. WAT distribution affects metabolic risk. Large amounts of white fat around the abdominal area is associated with a higher risk of metabolic syndrome (section 6), while fat in the hips and thighs does not.

2. Brown adipose tissue (BAT) or brown fat generates heat by burning calories, a process called thermogenesis. When it is cold, brown fat's lipid reserves are depleted, and its color gets darker. Brown fat may play a key role in keeping people lean (a person who is overweight has proportionally less brown fat than a person who is not overweight). Experiments have shown that adding more brown fat to mice has been found to increase the rate at which they burn energy, thus protecting them from diet-induced obesity.

Recent experiments have also revealed that brown fat's benefits go far beyond burning calories. A 2011 study using mice found that brown fat can fuel itself with triglycerides taken from the bloodstream—exactly the kind of fatty molecules known to increase the chances of developing metabolic syndrome.

Brown fat cells also draw sugar molecules from the blood, which could help lower the risk for type 2 diabetes; chronically high levels of blood glucose wreak havoc on the body's ability to manage those levels in the first place, which in turn sets the stage for diabetes.[12]

So brown fat is great; where do we get it? We're still working on that. But unless you want to spend hours sitting in icy bathwater, there is no comprehensive way to induce brown fat formation.

However, we have learned something cute:

Japanese White Mulberry (*Morus indica*)

Mulberries are the hanging fruit from deciduous trees that belong to the *Moraceae* family. Now, according to a study from China, this delightful fruit seems to contain a natural compound which will activate brown fat: rutin!

Study co-author Wan-Zhu Jin, Ph.D., of the Institute of Zoology at the Chinese Academy of Sciences, and team set out to investigate the metabolic effects of rutin, with the aim of determining whether the compound might aid weight loss.

Rutin acts as a 'cold mimetic' (pretending low temperatures) to activate brown fat.

For their study, the team added rutin (1 milligram per milliliter) to the drinking water of two groups of mice.

- One group of mice was genetically obese, while the other group had diet-induced obesity. Both groups of mice were fed the same diet throughout the duration of the study.
- In both groups of mice, rutin was found to activate brown adipose tissue (BAT), or brown fat, which led to increased energy expenditure, better glucose homeostasis—the balance of insulin and glucagon to maintain glucose levels—and fat reduction.

Additionally, the team found that rutin triggered the formation of brown-like fat cells in subcutaneous adipose tissue, the fat located under the skin, in both mouse models of obesity.[13]

May be time to get some of those mulberries and start munching!

It may also be that a mixture of quercitin and resveratrol (together, as opposed to just one or the other) can induce a change in white fat, turning it into the brown variety. Resveratrol, as we know, comes from red wine. The absorption of quercitin is known to be enhanced by red wine. Maybe these are reasons why the French are famously slim?[14]

PART 3. THE PLANS

FIND YOUR MOJO!

THE PLANS EXPLAINED

PART 3. THE PLANS

SECTION 14. **DIFFERENT DIETARY APPROACHES**

In this section, let's look at the numerous possible ways you can choose to lose weight...

First of all, let me caution you to ignore completely the opinions of "experts" and their ratings of diets, based on health and effectiveness. There are those—professors even—who have been peddling the fat myth for decades and will not back down and admit they were wrong. They remain in the Dark Ages of health care.

So we still hear, over and over, that the Atkins diet is "not safe"; it supposedly contains too much fat, which is "unhealthy". Yet the Atkins has been shown time and time again to perform (and outperform other diets), with oodles of great science. Still experts continue to downgrade it, because it is not supposed to work (it shouldn't work, in their limited estimations).

But it doesn't stop there. They can't spot a plan with dangers and difficulties, even if it's staring them in the face. One review I saw ranked the glycemic-index diet as a 3.5 (out of 5). Again, one of the proven plans, it works over and over, and for them it's a 3.5? No better than the powdered SlimFast approach, which they also rated 3.5! Huh?

The Slimfast plan does include one homemade meal daily, and the rest is powdered synthetic "fluff", but products are fortified, so the expert panel called it "mostly nutritious and safe." I call it dangerous, because it's synthetic (fake) and milk-based. Milk is about the worst food around and milk intolerance is rife everywhere. Whole races can't tolerate milk.

All of this is stupid: nitpicking over the amount of fat or calories, or whatever, and which diets are "healthy", and which supposedly not, all overlooks one vital point experts seem to miss or disregard altogether: *no diet, no matter how badly constructed, can be as dangerous as being seriously over-*

weight. So however unhealthy a diet in the short-term, it cannot but do good overall, if it gets the weight off.

Look, even to not eat at all is safe enough (starvation), if you don't go on for too long. In fact we are designed by Nature to suffer a bit of hunger and hardship now and then. I'll return to that theme later in the book.

Meantime, take my advice and choose your own diet plan. Whatever you feel comfortable with or works best for you (your own mojo). All that blather about lack of potassium, or not enough fiber, or too little carbohydrates, etc. etc. is of no relevance for a short-term get-the-weight-off program.

In this section I will quickly scan over the range of possibilities and what you need to look for.

Low Calorie Approach

Obviously, to a degree, all effective diets must have a certain amount of calorie control: Nutrisystem, South Beach Diet and so on. But this is something you can do by yourself, if you are willing to measure and count.

Almost everyone understands that eating fewer calories should lead to weight loss. What is not so well known is that, once you lose weight by this method, you will immediately re-gain the pounds as soon as you eat "normally" again.

A major disadvantage of this approach is that fats score high and so you are pressured to avoid fatty foods. That's a pity because we now know that eating fat and pushing it as far as ketosis is probably the very best way to lose weight (fastest, easiest and most permanent). In fact you may be able to lose weight for the first time by *increasing* your calorie intake by eating plenty of fats!

There is a myth perpetuated by those who want to make money from your struggles that "a calorie is a calorie; it doesn't matter where it comes from." That's just plain crazy and wrong. A sugar calorie behaves very differently once inside the body than a fat calorie, as we shall see.

But because of the constant emphasis on the concept of counting calories, more and more people over the last few decades have come to view the word "calorie" as a bad thing. This is unfortunate because calories are the fuel that power life. Without calories we'd be unable to move our muscles, develop brain cells, or function.

You can use these formulas to calculate a good estimate of the number of calories a man or woman would need during any given day:

- Adult male: 66 + (6.3 x body weight in lbs.) + (12.9 x height in inches) - (6.8 x age in years); or
- Adult female: 655 + (4.3 x weight in lbs.) + (4.7 x height in inches) - (4.7 x age in years).

Using such a formula will give you the number of calories you need each day to maintain your current weight. Obviously this approach makes no allowance for differences in activity levels.

You will need calorie counter tables, to look up the scores for different foods (at least at the outset, until you get used to what is low-calorie and what isn't).

Remember, not all calories are the same. Some come from foods that are nutrient dense, such as a piece of salmon or a cup of cooked greens, and some come from a slice of white bread with butter or a packet of candy. These latter are known as "empty calories" and are the kind to cut from the diet altogether.

The SAD, or standard American diet, is full of empty calories that come from foods high in added salt, sugar, and chemical ingredients. For example, the famous boxes of macaroni and cheese are not really nutritious, and are fattening and full of sodium. It would be better to get the same number of calories from a meal such as steamed fish, rice, and vegetables.

It is this last point that must be considered when you are about to begin a low calorie plan. The body uses the food we eat to create energy. These calories are either put to use right away, or stored for later use in the form of fat. When you eat more calories each day than you "burn", you put on weight.

Many low calorie plans do indeed allow you to quickly shed weight because you are, essentially, starving the body. Some will reduce the weight via "water weight" loss. Others send the body into what many feel is a "panic mode". This is a time when the body uses muscle for energy, and does not tap into any stored fat or calories. The body is tricked or confused and does not burn fat as a food resource but burns muscle. This shows up as uric acid in the blood (see ketogenic dieting, page 188).

For example, a small study in 2014 showed that losing weight too fast is more likely due to muscle loss, than getting rid of fat. Bad!

The researchers put 25 participants on a five-week very-low-calorie diet of just 500 calories per day. Another 22 volunteers went on a 12-week low-calorie diet of 1,250 calories per day.

At the end of the trial, both groups had lost about the same amount of weight (around 19 pounds). BUT, the weight loss on the very-low-calorie diet was mainly due to loss of muscle mass.

Put another way, muscle loss accounted for 18 percent of weight loss in the very-low-calorie diet group and just 7.7 percent of weight loss in the low-calorie diet group.[1]

Thus, the ideal low calorie plan is one that is not designed to force the body to rapidly shed many pounds. Instead, it is going to cut calories while providing complete nutrition. It will not lead to common side effects like fatigue, constipation, irritability, and digestive issues.

Don't fall for the claims that any low calorie plan is the easy answer to weight loss. It is usually advisable to drop no more than two pounds per week (after any initial loss of retained water weight in the first week of dieting). If you are eating in a way that causes you to lose five or more pounds per week, over the course of many weeks, you are likely to "bounce back" and re-gain that weight.

In general, low calorie diets are a bad idea (1/5).

Low Carbohydrate Plans

The original low-carb diet plan was invented by William Banting (1796 - 1878), who in 1863 published his booklet called *Letter on Corpulence, Addressed to the Public*, which contained the particular low-carb plan for the diet he followed. In the 1920s and 30s "Banting" was the word for slimming! It's a term you will still hear today.

The marvelous benefits of the low carb approach are twofold:

1. It's more natural (what humans as hunter-gatherers should be doing)

2. Many foods have zero score. That means you can eat as much of them as you like. No need to feel hungry! If you have a steak and artichoke fries and still feel unsatisfied, cook the whole meal again and eat it twice.

There are some very famous low carbohydrate plans available. These include Atkins, Paleo Diet and ketogenic dieting, among others. The fundamental concept behind all of them is the same, however, and that is that drastically reducing the amount of carbohydrate in the diet is going to lead to weight loss.

We have to eat something, so what do we eat instead? Fats! Fats are very satisfying to the appetite, which is the main reason you won't feel hungry using this approach. So another term for this method is the high-fat, low-carb approach (HFLC).

The emphasis is thus on meats, fish, plant foods and non-sugary drinks (even wine is allowed!)

Let's look aT the Atkins:

The Atkins Diet

This diet is so vast in scale, sweeping in social effect, and backed by solid medical science, that it is worthy of a section of its own. You might say that the "Atkins" is one of the benchmark standards for all slimming diets.

A lot of people are confused by the Atkins because of the controversy surrounding it. After all, some of its adherents insist that they consume vast quantities of bacon, sour cream, and red meat in order to keep their lean figures or to lose a lot of body weight. How, many wonder, could this high fat diet possibly allow someone to remain slim?

The answer is found in the process known as "ketosis" (section 14). To keep it as simple as possible, ketosis occurs when the body cannot use glucose in foods to create energy but must instead tap into any stored fats to do so.

Atkins eating consumes mostly protein, fat, and nutrient dense vegetable fiber. Carbohydrates are limited to the most minimal amounts and this allows the body to burn up the carbohydrate almost as soon as it is consumed. Doing this forces the body to start burning up stored fat for energy.

In contrast, let's say that you eat a baked potato, green salad, and piece of fruit at lunch time. This sounds like a healthy meal, but it is actually fairly high in glucose because of the number of carbs it contains. Your body would not burn fat to create energy after a meal like this because it would have all of the glucose it needed for a subsequent few hours' metabolism!

Fat would be the last thing used for energy when eating in this way and—even worse—any of the unused energy from that meal would be stored as fat.

The important thing is to ignore the bunk about saturated fats and how they are said to be "unhealthy". Firstly, we need saturated fats (our brains are over 50% fat) and we could not process our vitamins properly without fats: vitamins A, D, E and K are fat-soluble (meaning they are not easily absorbed with just water).

The truth is that fats kill the appetite and so are invaluable. But it's better than that: consuming plenty of fats puts us in a keto state and that means fast, effective weight loss!

More on this later.

Low carb diets: 5/5.

Glycemic Index Plans

Similar to, but not identical with, low carb eating is the glycemic index method. In this approach we are not just simply counting carbohydrates but taking a measure of how swiftly the particular foodstuff gets converted to blood sugar, if at all.

You will quickly see that cookies, for example—all sugar and refined white flour—or a scoop of chocolate ice cream, are likely to raise blood sugar levels almost immediately; within minutes in fact. Whereas a plate of sardines will have almost no effect on blood sugar.

The glycemic index (GI) is simply a tabulation of foods and how they affect blood sugar levels. So much so, that you won't get far using this method, unless you have a reliable published table of GI values for different foods.

The datum level for calculation is that of glucose itself, which is set at 100%.

Here are some examples:

FOOD	GLYCEMIC INDEX
Glucose	100
Potato	85
White bread	75
Sugar (sucrose)	68
Ice Cream	61
Bananas	52
Apples	38
Peanuts	14
Chocolate bar	40

Note that a banana has a higher GI than a chocolate bar!

The reader will readily see the need for actual tables. The complete list of the glycemic index and glycemic load for more than 1,000 foods can be found in the article: "International tables of glycemic index and glycemic load values: 2008" by Fiona S. Atkinson, Kaye Foster-Powell, and Jennie C. Brand-Miller in the December 2008 issue of Diabetes Care, Vol. 31, number 12, pages 2281-2283.

The master GI reference is considered to be the database maintained by Sydney University Glycemic Index Research Services in Australia. The database contains the results of studies conducted there and at other research facilities around the world.

Be aware that the scores are also affected by the *amount* of the food, so you will have to weigh everything. That sounds like a real chore but in fact you will soon get used to the scores and not need to weigh everything you eat!

Basically, a GI diet prescribes meals primarily of foods that have low values and strict avoidance of those foods which have the highest rating. Medium GI foods need to be eaten in controlled moderation.

Examples of foods with low, middle and high GI values include the following:

Low GI: Green vegetables, most fruits, raw carrots, kidney beans, chickpeas, lentils and bran breakfast cereals

Medium GI: Sweet corn, bananas, raw pineapple, raisins, oat breakfast cereals, and multigrain, oat bran or rye bread

High GI: White rice, white bread and potatoes

Commercial GI diets may describe foods as having slow carbs or fast carbs. In general, foods with a low GI value are digested and absorbed relatively slowly, and those with high values are absorbed quickly.

Results are often reported as somewhat variable. For example, a 16-year study that tracked the diets of 120,000 men and women were published in 2015. Researchers found that diets with a high GI from eating refined grains, starches and sugars were associated with more weight gain.[2]

Studies show that the total amount of carbohydrate in food is generally a stronger predictor of blood glucose response than the GI. So based on the research, for most people fighting diabesity, the best tool for managing blood glucose is carbohydrate counting, not using the GI.

GI Approach: 4/5

Meal Replacement Plans

Sometimes all you have to do is skip one meal and day and you will start to lose weight, even if slowly. If you were overweight but "in balance" as it were, then just slightly lowering your intake will begin the process of gradual weight loss.

For those who don't wish to skip a meal, or who lack the discipline to do so, then substituting one meal a day with a mix-and-swallow formula (usually a powder) is a possible solution.

The best-known meal replacement formula is the Slim Fast system. Originally just a powdered shake meal replacement, it has grown in popularity to the extent that its shakes come prepackaged in cans, and the line of products also includes meal bars and snack bars that can also work as substitutes.

This approach could work well if you want to drop no more than 20 pounds of fat. But the problem comes when you reach your target weight and resume "normal" eating. You don't want to put all the pounds back on again. Unfortunately, that is the common outcome of this approach, mostly because there isn't sufficient emphasis on nutritional education and lifestyle factors.

If you think about it for a moment, you will realize that the manufacturers of products such as these don't really want you to learn good habits. They want you to put back the weight and keep coming for the slimming product, time and time again. It's great for profits!

Apart from that, however, the program is relatively safe and easy. The shakes and bars are relatively low in sodium, high in fiber, and a good source for essential nutrients such as potassium, vitamin B-12, and vitamin D.

If using the Slim Fast diet, it's a good idea to take advantage of the online tools that they make available as well. This allows a dieter to start and track a plan, determine the most appropriate weight loss goals, and enjoy a host of tips that will provide them with some workable information.

Of course it needs saying that there are many current alternatives to the Slim Fast formula. Protein shakes abound and "meal replacements" is now a buzzword.

I have entered the field with my own high-quality, delicious protein meal-replacement shakes. These are not true milk shakes: there is no milk involved, although the formula does contain whey protein isolate...

Dr. Keith's Own® Protein Shakes come in a range of flavors, for variety and satisfaction: vanilla, chocolate and mocha. I can promise you that these formulas contain no GMO items, no soy, no sugar, no lactose, and are all natural (read the labels in future; the formulation may change from time to time).

Each serving is 180 calories but hopefully, by the time you have reached this part of the book, you won't worry too much about calories!

You can order these meal replacement shakes here: www.DrKeithsOwn.com/protein-shake

The Cambridge Weight Plan (formerly The Cambridge Diet)

Now we are moving towards more extreme restrictions of caloric intake.

The Cambridge Diet was the original 'meal replacement" weight loss plan. You didn't eat any food at all; just synthetically-formulated substitutes for ALL meals. It replaced eating with supposedly nutritionally complete, very low-calorie drinks and gave fast results.

It was developed in 1970 by Dr. Alan Howard at Cambridge University, England, and launched as a commercial product in the United States in 1980. The Diet was very popular in America but was also the subject of some controversy. It later came under scrutiny from regulators and health authorities after potential health concerns were raised. In the UK, the Cambridge Diet was launched in 1984. In 1986 the Diet was reformulated to adhere to recommendations made by the Commission on Medical Aspects (COMA).

You probably thought the Cambridge plan had vanished, when its founder Alan Howard died suddenly and at a tragically young age, whilst following his own regimen. It didn't do much to bolster public confidence in the safety of the plan.

The diet led to some cases of hospitalization and even death before Cambridge Plan International sought bankruptcy protection. The diet has also been linked to health complications like weakness, fatigue, irregular heartbeat and nausea.

However, it did survive the negative public relations impact and with a little dust down, a few slick platitudes and a complete makeover, it's back again, which is why I mention it here (I'm not recommending it though).

Meal Replacements: 2.5/5

Meals-To-Your-Door Plans

Examples: Jenny Craig, Nutrisystem.

The benefit of meals-to-your-door is that you don't have to spend time measuring, figuring out serving sizes, and ensuring that you are eating the appropriate amount of any specific food. This is one of the primary reasons that so many people like the Jenny Craig or Nutrisystem pre-packaged meals method.

These are, literally, no-brainers.

Rather than measuring out portions of pasta, vegetables, meats, etc. you simply get the meals delivered to your home and eat them "as is" or cook them according to directions. Some meals have the need for a green salad or side dish to be added, but that is usually the extent of the dieter's effort.

Jenny Craig clients can work with a consultant to discuss weight loss goals, lifestyle preferences, and even any specific food needs (such as vegetarian, kosher, allergies, etc.). From this discussion a unique plan is designed and started.

There are also specific levels in these programs, such as basic, premium and max (varies). This determines the foods you receive and the intensity or amount of exercise used for your plan. After that, you simply begin using the foods shipped to your home (with the usual addition of fresh fruits, vegetables, and some dairy). You get to choose the entrees and snacks sent each week, and you can enjoy a few desserts and even a cocktail or two now and then.

The benefits of this type of approach is that the meals are thought out for the client.

Typically, all dieters are kept within a 1250 calorie mark, and at 2300mg of sodium or less per day.

The main downside is that shipped meals are not fresh and make no allowance whatever for individual likes and, more importantly, individual food sensitivities or intolerances (section 5). In Nature a one-size-fits-all approach is doomed to failure and so it is with meals to the door plans.

The problem is that the "experts" designing the meals are ignorant dieticians, who know nothing of the science of weight loss, but simply follow official government scientists disastrously misleading guidelines (which is not the real expertise showcased in this book).

Moreover, cost can be a problem. Many people cannot afford to invest the money that it will take to succeed with this program, simply because it is essential to use at least a few weeks of the pre-packaged foods to get a good idea of actual serving sizes or portions (which is one of the main ways an approach like this helps the would-be dieter.

Meals to Your Door: 2/5

The Discipline and Accountability Methods

Example: Weight Watchers

Some weight loss programs do not rely on nutritional values and food composition. Weight Watchers, for example, although they publish recommendations and a point scoring system, mainly have their effect by making the individual accountable.

Someone who professes to want to lose weight and turns up at a meeting a week later not having lost a pound, feels somewhat foolish. If, indeed, he or she has gained weight in the meantime, shame is the likely emotion. This puts a certain pressure on the individual to conform.

Part of the Weight Watchers strategy is to work in a little "psychology". For example, when a human being feels as if they are deprived of something, such as sweet or tasty favorite foods, they are going to think a lot about those forbidden foods. This can lead to cravings and strong urges to consume them, and this can easily pressure the person to eat the forbidden food and go completely off their diet.

It's like, "Try not to think of an elephant." What's the first thing that leaps to mind when someone says this? A picture of an elephant, of course!

In principle there is something to be said for this allowance. But when the main problem for dieters is actual food addictions, breaking the grip of addiction altogether is much safer. Imagine treating a methadone addict by suggesting just a little of the forbidden drug now and again, "so you don't think about it." You know that's not a good strategy.

As I said, the main mechanism for Weight Watchers is accountability and a reliance on the natural human emotions of embarrassment and shame.

On the positive side, there is also the mechanism of pride of achievement. And also sociability and interaction with others engaged on a similar purpose.

Weight Watchers works for a lot of people. It's been around for decades. That must mean something!

Accountability: 2/5

The Lifestyle Approach

Here the emphasis goes beyond just what to eat and includes other lifestyle changes.

Examples: The Step Diet, Dukan diet

The Step Diet

If you have tried everything and you are looking for a totally novel way to lose weight, keep it off and become healthier, then the Step Diet could be for you. There's no counting of carbs, fat grams, or calories. In fact it's not really a diet as such, more of a lifestyle change. But it does change your eating habits and relates foods you eat to figures, so it definitely belongs in this book and is reviewed here, affectionately.

The Step Diet is one of the GREAT ways to slim.

The basic premise is simple: trade food for walking steps! Walk 10,000 steps a day and trim your portions by a quarter and you will lose weight, simple as that. Move more, eat a little less. If you want an ice cream, fine, but you have to walk the equivalent number of steps to work it off!

Brilliant!

Walking 10,000 steps per day for health and weight loss was popularized originally in Japan. But it isn't a magic number, or based on medical research; it's simply a good indicator of how active a person is.

Unless you have an active job such as a waitress or nurse, it would be difficult to log 10,000 steps just with daily activity. Most people achieve it by one or more sustained walks or runs, the equivalent of 30-60 minutes or more of walking per day.

The term Step Diet was developed in the USA by James O. Hill, John C. Peters, Bonnie T. Jortberg, and Pamela Peeke, for their book *The Step Diet*. It is a lifestyle program for both weight loss and weight maintenance. The easy-to-do plan helps dieters slowly increase their daily activity with the use of a pedometer. A pedometer (literally, a foot meter) is a small device attached to your waist belt or ankle and counts the click of bumps of every step you take (right foot – left foot = 2 clicks).

These days, most of us have a smartphone which will count your steps, more or less accurately, and log them, without the need for a pedometer.

Lead author James Hill, PhD, a well-respected obesity researcher, and co-founder of the US National Weight Control Registry (NWCR) and America on the Move, understands the importance of physical activity. He says you don't need to run marathons to control your weight, just strap on a pedometer and lace up a pair of sneakers and put one foot in front of the other.

If you're ready to make small adjustments in the way you eat, and if you want to start walking your way to weight loss, the Step Diet is a plan that has a lot to recommend it, because you will feel great, as well as look better.

What To Eat

Ready for this? You can eat whatever you like! Just cut back your usual portion size by about 25%. Then balance your daily intake with plenty of steps, starting at 2,000 and working your way up to 10,000 per day.

Healthy foods such as fruits, vegetables, whole grains, low-fat dairy, lean protein, and healthy fats are strongly encouraged but there are no forbidden foods. If you want to splurge on a piece of cheesecake, simply compensate with the appropriate number of steps.

Detailed charts for men and women are provided in the book, giving the number of steps needed to balance out the extra calories from your favorite foods. If you prefer other forms of exercise besides walking, there are charts showing the equivalent number of steps. For example, for women 150 steps can be traded for one minute of cycling.

Bottom line with the Step Diet, increase the number of steps you take throughout the day to increase energy expenditure and you will lose or maintain body weight.

Authors of the book argue that diets don't work because most are temporary solutions or quick fixes. The Step Diet is a health plan that shows you how to make small changes in eating and exercise habits that really do add up. Dieters are encouraged to take a hard look at their habits during the first week of the program. Then behavior tips throughout the book are designed to help you become more aware of eating mindfully and gaining control over your life problems.

On this plan you won't need to count calories or eat particular foods. The goal is to eat a healthy diet that satisfies hunger and results in slow and steady weight loss of 1 to 2 pounds per week. Emphasis throughout the book is on making small, permanent, easy changes in your diet and lifestyle that will promote a healthier energy balance.

Each 2,000-2,500 steps equals about a mile. Walking a mile burns about 80 calories for a 150-pound person. So if you want a 500-calorie treat, walk five miles and you're good! Enjoy the treat!

So How Much Is 10,000 Steps?

The key point to grasp is that we all clock up a number of steps each day, even without trying to exercise. Moving from the kitchen to the dining room, from the bedroom to the bathroom, from the house to the garage, all need a few steps and these add up.

If you are already logging 10,000 steps a day and not losing or maintaining your weight, then the key is to add another 2,000 steps per day (and/or eat fewer calories).

If that still doesn't work after a couple of weeks, add more steps or eat less. Eventually, this consumes too much time. Then you will need to increase your exercise intensity so more of your steps are brisk walking or jogging.

But seriously: if losing weight is such a problem, you need to be looking at things like low thyroid (section 11) or intestinal probiotics and pre-biotics (section 12).

How Long Can I Keep It Up?

Like any weight loss program, there is a start point and a finish. Once you get to the weight you want to be, then you slack off.

All successful programs allow you to shift gear and adapt what you have learned into a long-term healthy lifestyle. There should never be a finish to a diet plan; just a change of pace and rhythm, once you reach your ideal weight.

And so it is with the Step Diet. Once you reach your target weight (or during a pause), spend time adjusting and getting used to your new weight. Persist with your new habits and routines, with only a slight relaxing of the conditions, and learn to become the new healthy you!

The Step Diet authors point out that with all slimming plans, losing weight is the easy part. The tough part is keeping the lost weight off forever. On the Step Diet most weight loss occurs in the first 12 weeks, so from then on is a good time to get comfortable with your new weight and learn how to maintain it before going back on the program.

Lifestyle

What could be easier than walking more and cutting 100 - 200 calories every day? It's a shift anyone could make.

What I especially like about the Step Diet is that it is a whole-life change, not just food intake restrictions. OK, working off weight is harder than eating less, I made that point already. But there is that additional "feel good" factor from being more active.

After all, Nature designed us to walk freely through the forests and across prairies, or along the sea strand, never really stopping. We, as Homo sapiens, are itinerants and nomads; that's our biology. So any lifestyle plan which approximates to that is good.

Susan Finn, former president of the American Dietetic Association and chairwoman of the American Council on Fitness and Nutrition, loves the Step Diet. "It is one of the easiest strategies for weight loss -- all you need is a pair of sneakers, a pedometer and some simple guidance on proper portions and healthy eating behaviors to be successful," she says.

The fact is that The Step Diet cuts through all the clutter and scary science terms and makes losing weight or maintaining weight achievable for most everyone.

Remember, as I said earlier in the book, exercise isn't the quickest way to lose weight; but it's great for keeping the weight off.

You'll need the book, for all the advice, tips and tables in it. It's called The Step Diet and the book is packed with useful information. The biggest step you can take is to go buy the book and start pounding the highways or byways every day.

Step Diet: 4.5/5

The Dukan Diet

The diet developed by French slimming guru Dr. Pierre Dukan, has been much the rage at the time of writing. The Duchess of Cambridge chose to follow it, so an army of sheep did likewise! Still, that's no bad thing, since it's a good plan and rightly enjoys favor.

No sign of Cordon Bleu heavy cream and sauces here though! Dukan is a passionate believer that successful dieting is all about "rediscovering the pleasure" that comes with eating good food. His diet doesn't count calories but instead is based on high protein, low carb food intake (so nothing new there).

But exercise is an integral part of the diet and, to me, that's its main success "secret". The Dukan Diet program works in four sequential phases:

1. Attack phase (short sharp beginning): To kick-start weight loss, you are restricted to eating just protein for one to 10 days. You must also drink 1.5 litres of water and exercise for 20 minutes a day.

2. Cruise phase (settling in for the long haul): Alternate one protein day with a day of protein and non-starchy vegetables – so no potatoes – until you reach your desired weight.

3. Consolidation phase (making sure you never slip back): In addition to the protein-only meals and those with non-starchy vegetables, you may eat two slices of wholemeal toast a day, 40g of cheese and two servings of starchy foods per week. You can eat two "blow out" meals of your choice per week (he calls them celebration meals). No rules here, provided you return to the attack phase one day a week.

4. Stabilisation phase (creating new lifetime slimness): eat normally, but have just protein on one day a week and keep up the exercise.

It kicks off with an "Attack Phase". This is pretty tough: zero carbs, just protein items. There are 72 high-protein foods allowed including lean beef, chicken and fish without any added oil or butter. This phase lasts 5-10 days depending on your current weight and progress (something you measure from their "true weight calculator".

The main purpose of this first stage is to introduce good eating habits, while dealing with the usual diet hunger issues and breaking your addictions to sugar and starches. For most people this is also the phase with the biggest weight loss! As the time goes by your body will adjust to the new regime and lose weight at a more stable pace.

When You Reach Your Target Weight

I like the fact that Dukan thinks ahead and has answers for this very crucial moment. Normally, your body will be desperate to put back all the lost starvation reserves, as quickly as possible. You have to totally establish this "new you", otherwise you'll be a calorie sponge and bounce straight into the yoyo effect that so bedevils slimmers.

Dukan calls this the Consolidation Phase and it provides a crucially important period of transition between hardline dieting and a return to normal eating.

You'll need his book for further advice and instruction: The *Dukan Diet* (Crowne Archetype, New York)

Dukan and Similar: 4/5

Miscellaneous Diet Categories

There are a number of diets which have earned reasonable success rates. One is the DASH diet, beloved of orthodox doctors and scientists. It's published in the literature and does help control blood pressure, so it must be "correct"!

The DASH Diet

DASH is an acronym for "Dietary Approaches to Stop Hypertension". Though the ultimate goal of this diet is to reduce blood pressure by a few points each week, it is also a safe and moderately effective way to shed weight as well.

In a nutshell, the DASH Diet uses all kinds of foods, controlled portions, nutrient dense choices, and reduced sodium to create its results. It is similar to most of the weight loss programs designed for a maximum of one to two pounds per week, but it is not really meant to emphasize the weight issue.

Instead, those on the DASH Diet will work hard to reduce their daily sodium intake to levels that are far below the "norm". As an example, the typical person who eats commercial foods swallows more than 3000mg of sodium every day. This could be naturally occurring sodium in all food sources, plus added table salt or preservatives in food. If the typical person has no problems with hypertension or blood pressure, they can easily continue to consume this much sodium without many negative health issues.

However, those on the DASH Diet are seeking to decrease blood pressure by reducing sodium intake, and this means that no more than 2300mg will be allowed. There is even a lower level version of the diet that limits sodium intake to around 1500mg per day.

The diet is meant to provide up to 2000 calories per day, but can be easily adjusted to suit the BMR (basal metabolic rate) of the individual.

DASH dieting is not really a restrictive form of eating. Instead of eliminating any food groups (such as low carb dieting), this is a diet that emphasizes fruits, vegetables, whole grains, and low fat dairy. There are also servings of legumes, poultry, and fish in the diet, and even a small amount of red meat, sugar, and fat is included.

So one of the problems with this approach is individual food sensitivities. Having a little of everything means that nobody is safe from this effect!

In a way, DASH dieting is a tepid compromise that hardly ticks any of the boxes, never mind most of them. And allowing sugar in any quantity is foolish and ignorant.

Dash Diet: 3.5/5

The Mediterranean Diet

Although not a formally drafted diet or eating plan, and not typically recommended for weight loss, the Mediterranean diet has a lot to offer the would-be slimmer. It is more a way of life that is based on food patterns of the Mediterranean region (including Northern Africa and the Levant).

It can help an individual to improve their metabolic function, regulate their blood sugar, and reduce risks of many common and chronic concerns such as diabetes and heart disease.

It's largely plant based and is said to be low fat (arguable, if you have ever watched a Mediterranean chef pour on lashings of olive oil) and emphasizes vegetables, fruits, olive oil, legumes, fish, and unrefined cereals and grains. There is a bit of dairy in the plan, some bread, some wine, and only small amounts of meat. The best part is the taste: it's delicious.

As usual, there are supposed health "experts" who want to nitpick with this plan. For example, a lot of allowed foods are naturally salty (olives, cured cheese, salted anchovies, etc.) and therefore contain plenty of sodium. It's a totally misplaced objection.

Basically, this is a successful diet, by actual studies of healthy peoples in Italy, Greece, Spain and France. Corny dietician science is at a loss to properly explain why it works. It should NOT work is the official view.

However, the benefits are clear.

Mediterranean Diet: 4/5

The South Beach Diet

The South Beach Diet (SBD) is reviewed here, as just one example of a heavily commercialized "diet", of which there are a number on the market. Such systems make money (lots of money) and are more about commercial gain than optimum human needs. Just remember that... (be a little cynical for once!)

The SBD is one of the ones being heavily pushed by current TV advertizing. Of course throwing a lot of money at this kind of promotion is not proof the diet has real value. One woman (maybe an actress) saying "Trust me, it works" is not to the standard of scientific proof required.

So, is it beneficial? Like most diets, it works if you follow it. But is it easy to follow? That's a better question.

Often mislabeled a "low carb" diet, the South Beach Diet was actually created by a cardiologist who wanted to help patients to cut fat from the diet in a misguided and ignorant effort to reduce the risks of heart disease. However, the effectiveness of the plan in terms of weight loss soon brought it to the attention of the general public, and by the year 2000 it was a widely followed dieting program.

What makes the South Beach Diet different from many of the low carb plans is that it allows far more carbs into the daily program than any true low carb plan ever would. It simply eliminates the "bad carb" sources such as white flour, white rice, and white potatoes.

It cuts them because of their "GI" or glycemic index. In fact, the South Beach Diet is radically different from low carb eating because it does include most vegetables in the plan from the very beginning and then adds the brown rice and whole grain foods during later stages.

As just mentioned, this diet is done in "stages", and that is why many confuse it with low carb plans such as Atkins. However, where the other plans totally eliminate almost all sources of carbs, including huge lists of fruits and vegetables, the South Beach Plan does not.

This is because it is a plan meant to introduce someone to a new way of eating. This "new way" is simply one that emphasizes the good carbs and the good fats over the unhealthy ones.

The SBD Phases

Let's consider the three phases of the South Beach Diet to understand how it works.

In the first phase, the diet is very conservative. This is a period meant to help the dieter to alter their cycle of hunger away from the controls of sugar, processed foods, and high GI options. They will usually have to cut out sugar of any kind, fruit, the higher GI veggies, and all processed carbs for a two-week period.

At the end of this process they are going to transition into the more liberal second phase that is the weight loss phase. This goes on for as long as it takes for a dieter to reach their goal weight. It is a period in which whole grains, fruits, and veggies are allowed into the plan. After that comes the third phase, which is the ongoing phase of healthy eating for life.

Food Lists

Something that many people panic about is the elimination of fruit from the diet in the first phase. This is something that lasts for a total of 14 days, and after that, a long list of fruits is added including:

- Apples
- Bananas
- Blueberries
- Grapefruit
- Grapes
- Mango
- Oranges
- Peaches

People are advized not to drink fruit juices as these are extremely high in terms of GI (smoothies are better, since fiber and other food factors lower the overall sugar content).

Because the list of forbidden foods is much shorter than the list of foods allowed on the program, we'll give a quick review of what is cut from the diet in the first two phases.

Banned in Phase 1:

- Any starchy carbohydrate food - cereal, pasta, bread, potatoes, baked goods, and rice
- No alcoholic beverages
- No fruit or fruit juice
- No full fat cheese
- Any starchy vegetable - beets, carrots, sweet potatoes, yams, corn, or barley

Banned in Phase 2:

By the second phase, some of the forbidden items are added back to the list and the only forbidden foods are:

- White breads, pastas, rice, and similarly "white" starchy carbs
- No fruit juice, canned fruits, dried fruits, pineapple, and watermelon
- No full fat cream
- Starchy vegetables that includes beets, corn, and white potatoes

Dieting is for life (*Phase 3*) and that means shedding bad habits completely, not just giving up guzzles for a few weeks.

White flour, pastas, rice, potatoes and other starchy foods are bad choices and don't suddenly become magically healthy, just because you have reached your target weight.

Despite its shortcomings, the South Beach Diet is recommended by many professionals, because of its use of good fats and carbs, its customizable format, and its emphasis on nutritious foods.

It works if you do what they say but why sail close to the wind?

South Beach Diet (3/5)

Vegan and Vegetarian Diets

Let me state right at the outset that this section is not about whether animals have souls, or the morality of human exploitation of animals, or whether little furry beasts feel pain and anguish. I'm confining myself solely to the metabolic impact of different foodstuffs, in health and in sickness.

There is irrefutable evidence that anyone who follows a plant-based diet that is free of added sugar and salt, processed foods, and low in fat is likely to be quite thin. However, simply "going vegetarian" or even "vegan" will not necessarily help you to shed unwanted weight.

For clarity: a vegetarian is someone who does not eat the flesh of animals, such as meat, fish, and poultry, or any product for which an animal was hurt or killed (like calf rennet, used in most cheese-making), but will eat dairy products, eggs, and honey; whereas a vegan is someone who avoids any and all animal products and therefore does not even consume cheese, honey, dairy products of any kind, eggs, etc. A vegan diet consists entirely of plant-based foods such as fruits, vegetables, grains, oils, nuts, and seeds. Veganism is a stronger principle and many vegans will not even wear leather shoes.

While there are many vegetarians and vegans who are extremely thin (often underweight) because of their restricted dietary choices, there are also many vegetarians who are overweight as well. This is because they are using a lot of unhealthy options to ensure they get protein into their diets (grains particularly).

That's what we need to address. It is very hard being a vegetarian, not eating grains (which are carb-heavy), and even more difficult being a vegan. So very low-carb eating is OUT.

For example, the Atkins plan is one that most vegans and vegetarians would have a tough time following. That is because it uses fat and protein to generate energy rather than glucose from carbs.

This means that we have to consider other ways that a vegetarian or vegan eater can begin to shed some unwanted weight. The very first step would be to consider precisely what they needed in terms of daily caloric intake.

All human beings have a baseline number of calories that they require each day in order to maintain their current weight and to simply continue to function normally. The formula is given already on page 167.

Using the formula, you will come to a number which is actually the minimum number of calories you need every single day in order to just function. This means without making any caloric adjustment for exercise and activity levels.

Once a vegetarian or vegan understands the number of calories they require, they must develop a diet that will give them this figure. To realistically drop weight, he or she will have to create a deficit.

For example, the woman who needs to drop seven pounds should aim to lose one to two pounds per week. To do this would mean eating around 3500 to 7000 calories less than she actually needs. This would be done through a mixture of exercise and dieting.

One of the best tools to use is the GI index. It's not foolproof, as you have read, but the concern is to stop grains being converted quickly into glucose and so causing a sugar rush. Complex carbs are "slow carbs", whereas refined grains are definitely "fast grains" (high GI).

What are complex carbs? These are usually foods that are very high in fiber and which take the body a long time to digest and break down. They will often make us feel very full and satisfied with only a limited amount eaten, and they will take so long to digest that we are not hungry for a few hours and our blood sugar is not spiked. Complex carbs are usually, by their nature, nutrient dense and extremely beneficial.

Good examples include broccoli, spinach, beans and legumes, sweet potatoes, etc. These should comprise more than half of the carbs eaten by any vegetarian or vegan. When balanced in the diet and included in each meal, the vegetarian will be satiated and remain so for many hours.

Meals should always be a nice balance of these complex carbs with a bit of fat and protein at the appropriate percentages. I would recommend 15/20/65 for weight loss (15% carbs/20% protein/65% fats). You'll have to work hard to reach that proportion of fats: lots of coconut oil!

Here are some other fats and oils you can introduce (or emphasize more, if you already eat them): palm oil and cocoa butter (saturated); almonds, Brazil nuts and walnuts (monounsaturated); and tahini, an oily product made from sesame seeds. Don't overlook avocados, olive oil and soybeans, all of which have the kind of beneficial fat you want to incorporate into your nutrition plan.

Essential Fatty Acids (EFAs)

Crucial to human health are so-called essential fatty acids. The main ones of concern are DHA (docosahexaenoic acid) and EPA (eicosapentanoic acid). These quench inflammation and help weight loss. Unfortunately, both come almost exclusively from animal and fish dietary sources.

For vegetarians and vegans the important alternative option is ALA (alpha linoleic acid). Flax seed oil is rich in ALA. The body transforms ALA to DHA and EPA naturally. Unfortunately, a small percentage of individuals cannot make this conversion (a faulty gene). To avoid this concern, you can supplement with marine algae. This is one of the few direct ways to get plant-based DHA and EPA.

It's important because you can't properly lose weight, if you need to, without plentiful EFAs on hand.

Vegan (1/5), vegetarian (2/5).

(We should all eat more plant-based foods. But to eat only plant-based foods is contrary to Nature's workings. Hence the scoring.)

The Paleo or "Caveman" System

Now we are starting to get to the really good stuff!

In the 1980s I was one of a handful of doctors around the world pioneering an approach to food allergies using a "caveman" or Stone Age diet. Today we would call that paleo eating, paleo being the word for very old, in the archeological sense. My name became so firmly associated with this type of diet in the 1980s that the BBC and other media sources christened me "The Stone Age Doctor"!

Think of what a Stone Age human (Neanderthal or Cro-Magnon) walking through the forest would be eating: a little meat when lucky, fish (when lucky), gathered roots and vegetables, fruits (when in season) and he would drink water only.

That pretty well sums up paleo-style eating.

The dieter is, in effect, avoiding the modern foods, that are not part of our biological heritage: no cereals (grains), cattle and dairy produce, alcohol, sugar, tea, coffee and manufactured derivative foods.

The dieter will consume a diet that is high in healthy fats: fatty fish, and lean meats. These are foods that contain large quantities of omega-3 fatty acids, and this is good for the brain and the body. Omega-3s are also very anti-inflammatory.

No salt or sugar and especially no "flavorings" (MSG etc.), thought natural herbs are just fine.

Contrary to popular belief, Paleolithic humans ate enormous amounts of plant material. He or she was ambulant most of the time, thus consuming a lot of calories, and the hidden benefit of this is that anti-oxidants and other nutrients in plant food were actually consumed in quite large quantities.

From evidence found in campgrounds and middens (waste dumps, which give us clues to lifestyle, such as animal bone, human excrement, botanical material, mollusc shells, pottery, and other artifacts associated with past human occupation), we can reconstruct the diet of Stone Age Humans accurately.

Excavations reveal what is called a hunter-gatherer diet. That means someone who hunts and gathers, obviously. Our story books put a lot of emphasis on the hunting activities of our ancestors but actually women gathered around 60% of calories eaten (presumably while the men sat around the fire and talked about past hunts or future excursions!) Gathering foods would mean fruits, nuts, berries, seeds, roots and shoots.

In other words, our ancestors ate and drank foods limited to meats, fish, fruits and vegetables (roots and berries). They drank only water, or sometimes blood. Of course this does not sit well with current vegetarian propaganda, that our teeth are of the herbivore pattern, but facts are facts. The middens do not lie.

You will try to enjoy a large amount of seasonal produce. Paleolithic humans followed their food sources. That means they ate the available vegetables and fruits. You also get to enjoy the bounty of the season, with very few items "off limits". The usual rule is no potatoes, corn, or beans, as these were not foods that any Paleolithic human would encounter. You will instead eat nuts, seeds, oils, and even avocados as these are considered "valid" food sources.

You will feel full. Very few people eating Paleo-style experience true hunger pangs. Instead, you will start to feel much more satisfied than you have in the past because you are consuming so much fiber, drinking so much water, and eating high amounts of nutrients and "good fat". Plus there are no addictive carbs in paleo eating.

So you can expect to lose weight quickly and easily with the paleo system. It depends how strict you are. Some paleo cookery sites, for example, propound the use of honey and maple syrup as suitable for sweetened "paleo-style" desserts. It's true that Stone Age humans would occasionally have the pleasure of delicious honey. They probably also occasionally had rotted fruits turned to alcohol. That must have been a pleasant surprise for them.

But really, eating or drinking such foods on a daily, or even weekly basis, is not truly natural. Better to be strict and avoid such luxuries. You want to re-train your palate to manage without sweeteners and booze. You'll lose weight faster if you do.

I urge you to forget everything you read or hear about the dangers of "red meat". I put that term in quotes because I have never seen a study that looked at red meat. All of them are contaminated by the fact that researchers always want to include meat derivatives, as if that were just the same thing.

So "read meat" studies, include offal, sausages, cured meats, smoked products (which are not usually smoked but chemically flavored) and other adulterated meat sources.

To just label these "red meat" is an adulteration of science.

No matter who you are, you will shed some weight when eating according to the rules of the Paleo Diet. This is an optimal way of eating for the human body. It is a diet designed to make our bodies fat burning machines and yet to deliver amazing amounts of nutrition. It is one of my top-recommended diets.

Disadvantages: Not many really. Bad breath can occur, especially if you go ketotic, as with the Atkins Diet. Drinking plenty of water can help and chewing sugar-free gum. Just be aware that sugar-free means some synthetic substitute is used instead.

Constipation is a big issue for many. Lack of vegetable and grain fiber is a significant factor in this. It will eventually sort itself out, as the body becomes accustomed to the newer regimen.

A note for vegans and vegetarians. To eat paleo you will need to substitute meat and fish with other proteins:

- Hemp protein
- Spirulina
- Rice protein
- Pea protein
- Vegan protein

Paleo Dieting: 5/5

The Ketogenic Principle

The "Keto Diet" is sweeping the world right now. For one simple reason: it works! But it's not a fad. The US government official "food pyramid" is the real fad diet! It's only been around a few decades and has proved itself disastrous for anything but gaining weight and falling sick.

The keto principle, on the other hand, has been the way humans ate for a million years or more! The so-called hunter-gatherer diet is essentially ketogenic, meaning plenty of fats and few, if any, carbs. Plus there were periods of fasting or starvation, alternating with an abundance of food. It would depend on how successful the hunting and gathering was, of course. This ebb and flow of food is crucial to Nature's way. More of that when we come to intermittent fasting.

Let me explain ketosis.

It means a state of unfamiliar metabolism in which the body is supplied with little or no carbohydrate and so is forced to burn fat to create energy. All very low carbohydrate programs are essentially ketotic, when pushed to the full, so this approach is integral to the Atkins plan, paleo eating and the 500-calorie HCG diet (see page 193)

Deliberately inducing a ketotic state (the keto diet) has been used clinically for around a century. In the 1920s it was used as a therapy for seizures in children and helped in at least 50% of cases (in my view that's likely due to avoidance of grains, which are highly inflammatory).

More recently a high-fat, low-carb regimen (HFLC) has been used for such diverse conditions as epilepsy, obesity, diabetes, cardio-vascular disease, cancer, auto-immune diseases and dementia (though again, I'd like to suggest that allergy avoidance is at least a significant aspect of the undoubted clinical successes; see section 5).

The body maintains a small store of carbohydrates, as glycogen within the liver, sufficient to supply blood glucose for only 24 – 36 hours. Once this store is exhausted, the body turns to its backup source of energy: fat deposits. Burning up fat leads to a residue of substances we call ketones: betahydroxybutyric acid, acetoacetic acid and acetone. These substances are responsible for the sickly-sweet breath smell of someone in a ketotic state.

With a ketogenic diet you will change several health parameters for the better. Blood glucose will fall dramatically, insulin resistance decreases and soon vanishes and you will lose weight, obviously. But you will find a surprise bonus: you feel alert, energetic, brightly focused and NO HUNGER! The human brain likes ketones; in fact it flourishes using ketones for energy—much more so than burning glucose for energy.

Also, the heart works more efficiently when using ketones for energy.

Finally, one other surprise benefit: according to a study published in Nature magazine (January 2014) you will quickly switch your bowel flora to the right sort with keto dieting (more bacteroides, less firmicutes strains. See section 12)[3]

How Do I Keto?

Comparing paleo eating to keto eating, the principle difference is in the proportion of fat. Whereas paleo would typically be 40/30/30 (40% of calories from fat; 30% from protein; 30% from carbohydrates—give or take): for ketogenesis to work, you'll need up to 70% of your calories from fat; 20% from protein; and only 10% from carbs.

So we have to eat a lot of fats. That's good, because it kills the appetite. Forget all the propaganda about dietary fats, unsaturated fats, polyunsaturates, cholesterol and the rest of it. Healthy (non-trans) fat is good. It is the slimmer's friend!

Ways to crank up your fat intake includes things like "bullet-proof" coffee (regular coffee with melted coconut oil and/or butter, instead of milk).

Other foods to go for include:

Salmon and other fish which are rich in B vitamins, potassium and selenium, yet virtually carb-free. So-called oily fish (salmon, sardines, mackerel, etc.) are high in omega-3 fats, which have been found to lower insulin levels and increase insulin sensitivity in overweight and obese people.

Low-carb (non-starchy) vegetables. Most vegetables contain very few net carbs but "starchy" vegetables like potatoes, yams or beets are high in carbs and are best avoided.

Low-carb veggies make great substitutes for higher-carb foods. For instance, cauliflower can be used to mimic rice or mashed potatoes; "zoodles" can be created from zucchini; and spaghetti squash is a natural substitute for spaghetti. Wholefoods Markets even produce a butternut squash "spaghetti" which is delicious and really does the job for you Italiano-philes.

Cheese is both nutritious and delicious. There are hundreds of types of cheese. Fortunately, all of them are very low in carbs and high in fat, which makes them a great fit for a ketogenic diet. Beware of dairy allergies. Mostly this isn't a problem, even to those with milk intolerance. You can always try goat and sheep cheese as alternatives (chèvre, manchego, roquefort, sheep and goat ricotta, etc.)

Cheeses contains conjugated linoleic acid, which is a fat that has been linked to fat loss and improvements in body composition.

Avocados. Avocados are incredibly healthy. Hess avocados have a reputation for benefitting cancer. In addition, avocados may help improve cholesterol and triglyceride levels.

Avocados contain 10% fat, half of which is monounsaturated (like olive oil).

In one study, when people consumed a diet high in avocados, they experienced a 22% decrease in "bad" LDL cholesterol and triglycerides and an 11% increase in "good" HDL cholesterol.

Meat and Poultry. It's best to choose grass-fed meat, if possible. That's because animals that eat grass produce meat with higher amounts of omega-3 fats, conjugated linoleic acid and antioxidants than meat from grain-fed animals. Grain-fed animals can even carry over the allergen, so corn allergic patients may react to corn-fed chicken.

Eggs. Eggs have been demonized for decades. You still see egg whites offered as the "healthy" alternative. But ask yourself: which part of the egg contains the nutrients that enable a healthy chick to grow and multiply in size, over and over? The yolks of course, the only worthwhile part of the egg. The whites are just junk; padding to protect the chick from damage. Useful for the chef but not for your cells!

Virgin Coconut Oil. VCO is one of the most perfect keto companions; it's healthy and nutritious. To begin with, VCO contains a mixture of lauric acid and medium-chain triglycerides (MCTs). Unlike long-chain fats, MCTs are taken up directly by the liver and converted into ketones or used as a rapid source of energy.

In fact, coconut oil has been used to increase ketone levels in people with Alzheimer's disease and other disorders of the brain and nervous system.

It's great for weight loss. In one study, men who ate 2 tablespoons (30 ml) of coconut oil per day over a 12-day period lost 1 inch (2.5 cm), on average, from their waistlines without making any other dietary changes.[4]

Plain Greek Yogurts, Quark and Cottage Cheese. Plain Greek yogurt and cottage cheese are healthy, high-protein foods, but essentially low-carb, high fat (LCHF). Add nuts, cinnamon, berries, etc. for a tasty keto snack.

Extra-Virgin Olive Oil. EVOO provides impressive benefits for your heart, as well as weight loss. It is an essential component of the Mediterranean diet (maybe THE component that does all the good). It is the ideal base for salad dressings (vinaigrette) and mayonnaise.

EVOO is high in antioxidants known as phenols. These compounds further protect heart health by decreasing inflammation and improving artery function.[5]

Nuts and Seeds. These diet-friends are healthy, high-fat and low-carb foods. Frequent nut consumption has been linked to a reduced risk of heart disease, certain cancers, depression and other chronic diseases. Furthermore, nuts and seeds are high in fiber, which can help you feel full and absorb fewer calories overall.[6]

Berries. Most fruits are too high in sugar to include on a ketogenic diet, but berries are an exception. Berries (raspberries, strawberries, blueberries) are very low in sugar and high in fiber.

Butter and Cream. Obviously good to include on a ketogenic diet and, like other dairy products, butter and cream are rich in conjugated linoleic acid, the fatty acid that may promote fat loss.

Shirataki Noodles. Shirataki noodles come in a variety of shapes, including rice, fettuccine and linguine. They can be substituted for regular noodles in all types of recipes. These are a fantastic addition to a ketogenic diet. They are very low carb (less than 1 gram of carbs per serving) and only 5 calories, because they are mainly water! (see page 149).

Dark Chocolate and Cocoa Powder. Finally, a real treat! Cocoa has been called a "super fruit," because it provides at least as much antioxidant activity as any other fruit, including blueberries and acai berries. In fact Prof. Norman Hollenberg from Harvard Medical School declared that epicatechin from chocolate was so valuable as a health-booster that it ought to be considered a vitamin.

Somewhat surprisingly, chocolate can be part of a ketogenic diet. However, it's important to choose dark, unsweetened chocolate that contains a minimum of 70% cocoa solids, preferably more.

So you see, there are plenty of foods to choose from. And, it needs to be said, you can break out once in a while. You don't have to strictly adhere to keto-friendly foods, providing you know your keto status.

One of the best ways to measure that is to get yourself a keto meter; preferably one that measures glucose levels too (see below).

Signs You Are In Keto

You will pretty soon become familiar with certain feelings that tell you everything is going great.

1. Bad breath. This is due to the actual ketones, which smell somewhat like aircraft dope (betahydroxybutyric acid, acetoacetic acid and acetone).

2. Weight loss (of course!)

3. Increased ketones in the blood (measured by a meter)

4. Urinary ketones (you can buy urinary ketostix—but these are not as accurate as blood monitoring).

5. Appetite suppression.

6. Increased clarity and focus.

7. Fatigue at certain times. You may feel more energetic some of the time. But there will also be times when you seriously want to sit down and take it easy.

8. Temporary insomnia. It affects you when you first start. The brain has to switch over from glucose metabolism for energy to burning ketones. This can take a little time but persist anyway. The brain actually prefers ketones as fuel, once it has made the switch.

Keto Flu

Now here's an odd thing. People who switch to keto dieting often experience strange, unwanted symptoms that mimic a viral attack. So it's been christened "keto flu".

Typically, there are aches and pains, dizziness, bad breath, constipation, fatigue and feeling generally unwell. It's NOT flu of course, and is not a problem; you'll still lose weight. It's just one of things you have to work through (like a detox).

It happens while you are switching from a sugar dependent state to a fat adapted state. That's when the body produces less insulin, because it's increasingly redundant.

As my friend Graham Simpson MD points out (*The Metabolic Miracle*), this transition is weird and sometimes uncomfortable, because we have in a sense lost our historical and biological connection to ketone bodies, due to eating too many unnatural carbs.

Testing For Ketosis

I remarked that Robert Atkins' diet works as a high-fat, low-carb approach. Many patients reach a ketotic state and indeed this was flung at Atkins as a serious potential danger of his method; all nonsense and ignorance, of course. The ketosis state I am describing has nothing to do with the state of ketoacidosis, a dangerous complication of diabetes.

Atkins himself never measured blood ketones, though in latter years he did turn to measuring urinary ketones. But we can do better. Today—thanks to the current keto craze—there are numerous online sources of keto blood testing equipment. You can purchase a small kit from Amazon for between $50 and $100 which will enable you to monitor your level of ketosis on a frequent basis. I chose the Keto-Mojo, which measures blood glucose as well as ketones, but that's not a recommendation. Just a fact.

Are such devices worth it? Obviously it's easy to eat HFLC without one. This is for those fixated individuals who want definite proof that they are eating so little carbs that insulin levels are low and fat burning is maximized.

If you get one, aim for a ketone level somewhere between 1.5 – 3. That would be an optimal level for maximizing weight loss. It also tells you that insulin levels are satisfyingly low.

It is a useful tool if you are serious about managing a ketotic state. There are a number of ways that you can fail to get into ketosis. A blood ketone meter may give you a disappointing result but at least you can start looking for foods which interfere with the keto effect.

Keto Diet: 5/5

The HCG Method

To complete this section on keto dieting, I call everyone's attention to the success of the approach known as HCG diet. It uses a 500-calorie limitation, which is clearly below the levels needed for keto dieting. The trick is to use HCG to kill the appetite. Of itself, HCG has no weight-loss properties; it's the low-calorie eating which produces the weight loss.

This is more than a diet; it includes the taking of a specific hormone supplement, designed to trick the body into losing weight. I call it a weight loss therapy, rather than a diet. As originally developed, it was a medical specialty protocol, using injections of real **h**uman **c**horionic **g**onadotrophic (HCG), to fool the body into believing it was pregnant. More of why that is an advantage in just a moment. And before you ask, yes, it does work for men, even though we do not tend to get pregnant!

Today, the vast majority of the marketers and adherents of the HCG plan use a homeopathic version of the hormone, which is cheaper, probably safer and can be self-administered. I will not be going into the controversy over the validity of homeopathy in these pages. Suffice it to say that there are millions who have successfully tried this approach and it is probably one of the five-star plans, if done properly.

I myself experimented with it a few years ago and lost a satisfying 28 pounds in just 30 days. The only possible negative is that my wife was convinced that my personality changed, while taking the homeopathic HCG. She's usually right, so be warned (men, especially).

Here's the story...

The use of HCG injections coupled with an extremely low calorie diet was pioneered in the 1950s by a British endocrinologist, Dr. A T W Simeons, working in Rome. He proved that when both the correct amount of HCG was administered and his food plan was followed as he had designed, both males and females had the ability to lose extraordinary amounts of abnormal fat in relatively short periods of time. More than with just diet and exercise alone.

HCG is a hormone that is produced by the embryonic chorion during pregnancy. Its presence is a signal that implantation in the womb has taken place and that the woman's metabolism will henceforth be subjugated to that of the fetus' requirements. So, when the calorie intake drops to 500 per day, as is prescribed in this therapeutic regimen, the body is used as an alternative emergency food supply, for the "fetus" that does not exist.

The body burns fat at a great rate and, effectively, turns this from a 500 -calorie diet into probably around 1500 calories. As a result, fat is consumed but the patient does not feel hungry. The patient is eating his or her own fat tissues. Brilliant!

And that's the answer to silly fools who say, "HCG has been tested and proved not to work for weight loss". It doesn't cause weight loss on its own; it's the 500-calorie diet that brings about the weight loss. Nobody can eat so few calories and fail to lose weight very quickly. But such a person would be extremely miserable, with low energy and continuous griping hunger.

The magic here is that the HCG takes away the hunger by letting the slimmer feed on their own body fat.

Nevertheless, it is best to follow Simeon's principle of 2-day initial "loading"; that is, eating a lot of food in a short time, so you feel stuffed. Then when the 500-calorie days kick in, you have a little momentum going, and will feel less hungry.

Recommended durations are a 30-day spell, followed by a rest interlude; or a 45-day spell, if you can hack it and provided you are under skilled medical care. Never go on for longer periods. Take breaks and then resume; it is the safest way to do this.

Homeopathic HCG began being successfully used around 2008 by many Naturopathic Professionals as an alternative to HCG prescription injections. However, shortly thereafter, a major manufacturer of homeopathic HCG allowed lay people to purchase the product direct and sell to anyone without the necessary professional knowledge and experience needed to oversee the plan safely. That incident was the start of the rampant, uncontrolled, non-regulated selling of homeopathic HCG products on affiliate marketing websites, e-Bay, Amazon and the likes.

Coupled with blatant false claims copied from Kevin Trudeau's book *The Weight Loss Cure*, the HCG diet again has come under severe censure and criticism.[7]

Don't make the controversy worse. Stay completely away from websites selling this as snake oil and hokum. Just do it quietly and under the radar, by yourself, working with a real licensed practitioner, to ensure your safety and prevent HCG diet therapy from being banned altogether.

HCG Diet: 4.5/5

Quick and Simple Diet #5. Eat More Slowly

By investigation, overweight people eat faster than normal weight or underweight people, that's the conclusion of a 2011 paper, presented at The Obesity Society annual meeting, Orlando, Fla. Thing is: does it mean anything?

It might seem logical to jump to the conclusion that those who eat faster, eat more in a given time and therefore put on weight.

But the study also found that men eat faster but there is no evidence that men are more persistently overweight than women. Indeed, ordinary common sense suggests it's the other way round.

We are always being told to eat more slowly and enjoy our food more, as an adjunct to weight loss, and that makes sense. But it doesn't follow that those who eat more quickly necessarily eat more; it depends on how much they put on their plate. Quick eaters may just finish first and may not feel they have to ask for seconds, like Oliver Twist!

Seeking insight into the role that eating rate plays in quantity of food consumed, researchers from the University of Rhode Island also saw that refined grains -- found in white breads, pastas and potatoes -- are eaten faster than healthier whole grains.

According to author Kathleen Melanson, director of the university's Energy Balance Laboratory, it was obvious that there was a marked gender difference. Part of it might be that men have larger mouths, but it also might be related to higher energy needs. Another possibility could be related to social norms -- women may feel they have to eat slower.

Melanson, also an associate professor of nutrition and food science, said she was pleased that the research also validated that those who claim they are fast or slow eaters are generally accurate in their assessment.

In one study, Melanson and her team found that fast eaters consumed about 3.1 ounces of food per minute, medium-speed eaters ate 2.5 ounces per minute, and slow eaters consumed 2 ounces per minute. In calories: men ate about 80 calories per minute, while women downed about 52 calories per minute.

Interestingly, the men who called themselves slow eaters ate at about the same rate as the women who said they were fast eaters.

The second study found a close link between eating rate and body mass index (BMI), with those with higher BMIs typically eating considerably faster than those with lower BMIs. (BMI is a calculation based on height and weight: see page 32) The researchers also observed that participants eating a meal of whole grains -- whole-grain cereal and whole-wheat toast -- ate significantly slower than those eating a similar meal made of refined grains.

Presumably this is because whole grains require more chewing and also, because digestion starts in the mouth, if you have something highly processed, it doesn't take as much to digest that... whereas whole grains take a lot more to start breaking down.[8]

PART 3. THE PLANS

SECTION 15. THE BEST, EASIEST AND FASTEST METHOD WE HAVE

OK, early on I promised you I would point you towards the best (fastest, easiest and most sustainable) method of weight control—something backed by all the best of current science and even archeological evidence. Here I am now delivering on that promise!

In fact its nature's own way, programmed into our genes! I'm talking about the technique we call *intermittent fasting* (IF). We don't specify so much which foods you should eat but rather when you should eat them. But the diet will bite hardest and you'll lose weight much quicker if you couple it with keto or paleo eating.

In fact keto or paleo means high fat, low carb eating (HFLC) and that really helps by eliminating hunger. The more fat you eat, the more satiated you feel.

IF is not a diet in the conventional sense but more accurately described as an eating pattern, that cycles between periods of fasting and eating. It's currently very popular in the health and fitness community.

Fasting has been a pattern throughout human evolution. Ancient hunter-gatherers didn't have supermarkets, refrigerators or food available year-round. Sometimes they couldn't find anything to eat. As a result, humans evolved to be able to function without food for extended periods of time.

So IF is actually nature's way. You cannot go wrong if you follow her precepts. You can't be unhealthy if you eat naturally and that means you can't be overweight!

Intermittent Fasting Methods

There are several different ways of doing intermittent fasting — all of which involve splitting the days or weeks into eating and fasting periods. During the fasting periods, you eat either very little or nothing at all. Just a handful of nuts, a slice of ham, celery and peanut butter...

Of course it means you are almost guaranteed to be keto on your fast days. That means you'll burn up fat like a furnace. You'll pull fat from your liver and burn that. Fat from round your heart and other organs and burn that.

The big surprise is that you really don't feel hungry. It seems strange. But if you remember that hunger is more to do with carb withdrawals than actual need of food, then it starts to make sense.

In fact fasting will turn OFF your ghrelin hormone and so you don't feel hungry. That's a promise (but if you do, early on, just eat a half dozen cashews or some ham).

There are several ways to do an intermittent fast:

The 16/8 method (also called the Leangains protocol) means just fasting for 16 hours a day. You have an 8-hour eating window to match, say 10.00 am to 6.00 pm or 1.00 pm to 9.00. It depends on your work routine. Outside those 8 hours, just don't eat! That's not so difficult. But it does mean you must stop mindless eating and nibbling.

Many people find the 16/8 method to be the simplest, most sustainable and easiest to stick to. It's also the most popular.

5/2. A little tougher is doing a 2-day fast every week. That 2 days on and 5 days off.

1/1. You can do day on, day off, if you are in a hurry to lose weight. Eat well on your meal days though. I have already pointed out you'll lose more muscle mass than fat if you go too quickly. This one is a bit close to the wire.

30/5. Fasting 5 days in every month. 5 days in a row is tough but some people enjoy "getting it over with". Whether or not it suits you to do it this way is just a matter of temperament. There's no difference between any of these IF patterns.

Best not to eat at all on the fast days (200 calories or less) but the published 5-2 or "Fast Diet", attributed to Dr. Michael Mosley, allows you to consume 500–600 calories on the fast days.

It goes without saying that you don't try to compensate for the fast days by guzzling and gorging on the allowed days! Just eat sensibly and enjoy the best of the foods you would normally eat. You've been taught enough about food in these pages to make sensible choices.

You may need to re-read the sections on paleo eating and the ketogenesis diet; these are crucial. Paleo eating, or Stone Age eating, as I have already explained, is our true biological way of life.

There were no "farmer foods" such as cereals or dairy products. Eggs and honey would be very rare, and seasonal. So you can see the pattern here. Definitely no sugar, no milky tea or coffee lattes and capuccinos (drink it black, or not at all), absolutely no breads, cookies, cakes or pies! Alcohol would be a rare and providential accident, in which a band or tribe stumbled across a supply of partially fermented (rotted) fruits. Again, very seasonal.

Not a trace of the "scientifically-based" stupid food pyramid that was foisted on us for over 40 years, note! Instead of eating 60 - 70% carbs, as we are told, the correct ratio for humans is about 70% fat, 20% protein, and only about 10% from carbohydrates.

But the really important quality of Stone Age eating was the pattern, rather than the content. Food would be very intermittent. Exercise was almost continuous. So to closely copy the eating habits of the time we should keep moving and take food only intermittently. The desire to stuff our mouths hour after hour is completely contrary to what nature intends us to do.

That's why eating by the clock, the "now it's lunchtime" mentality, gets us to overeat substantially. We are conditioned to eat three meals a day, because that's what we have always done and what almost everyone else does! We need to break this tyranny.

Two important qualifiers: when I say fasting, it does not mean not even a crumb in your mouth. You can nibble nuts, grapes, ham or some cheese. You can even down a couple of glasses of wine (2 glasses for men, 1 glass for women). It will not hamper your results. Just make sure you are 200- 300 calories or less, so that intake is "unimportant".

On your non-fast days, stick to keto or at least paleo.

The Mosley Fast Diet (also known as The 5:2 Diet)

You may also come across it called the Mosley Diet or the 5-2.

It's a much gentler version of the intermittent strict fasting I have just described. The concept is simplicity itself: fasting is tough but you have to do something to lose weight. So, fast gently some days and eat normally on others; the question then is just the ratio of eating days to fasting days.

It all started with a documentary by British TV host and doctor Michael Mosley (a sort of British Dr. Oz), who experimented with intermittent fasting to see if it helped him lose weight and feel better.

He started out with a full fast and eventually, after trial and error, arrived at a ratio that worked for him: 2 days of partial fasting interspersed with 5 days of normal eating. The result: 20 pounds lost in nine weeks, along with a drop in cholesterol and blood sugar levels.

When his TV program *Eat, Fast, and Live Longer* aired on the BBC in August 2012, it was an overnight sensation.

Cutting calories in this way may reduce levels of a potentially-dangerous hormone IGF-1 (insulin- like growth factor 1) in the blood. Previous research has found that a drop in the blood level of IGF-1 triggers the body to turn on cellular repair mechanisms, protecting itself against cancer, heart disease, and other fatal illnesses.

It may also be that intermittent fasting significantly increases insulin sensitivity, aiding blood sugar regulation. We know that the lower insulin levels you can get, the longer you'll live.

IF also stimulates stem cell activity, which is great for repair and living longer.

So! Lots of benefits with this approach, in addition to just dropping the pounds!

The 500 calories is not a true fast, of course. It's also strangely reminiscent of what A T W Simeons evolved for his HCG diet, don't you think? It's too tough to do every day but even the hardened food addict can usually manage to eat less two days a week.

Intermittent Fasting: 5/5

PART 4. THE REST

BEYOND THE PLANS

PART 4. THE REST

SECTION 16.
BARIATRIC SURGERY

Bariatric surgery (weight loss surgery) includes a variety of procedures performed on people who are obese. Sometimes incorrectly spelled baryatric, the word comes from the Greek words "baros" meaning "weight or pressure" (as with a barometer for air pressure) and "iatrikos" meaning "medicine".

Weight loss is achieved by a number of procedures, including reducing the size of the stomach with a gastric band (reversible) or through removal of a portion of the stomach (not reversible) or by resecting and re-routing the small intestines to a small stomach pouch (gastric bypass surgery).

The U.S. National Institutes of Health recommends bariatric surgery for obese people with a body mass index (BMI) of 40 or more, and for people with a BMI of 35 and serious coexisting medical conditions such as diabetes.

However, research is emerging that suggests bariatric surgery could be appropriate for those with a BMI of 35 to 40 with no comorbidities or a BMI of 30 to 35 with significant comorbidities. [1]

A medical guideline by the American College of Physicians concluded that surgery could be justified as a treatment option for patients with a BMI of 40 kg/m2 or greater who instituted but failed an adequate exercise and diet program (with or without medication) and who were suffering obesity-related comorbid conditions, such as hypertension, impaired glucose tolerance, diabetes, hyperlipidemia, and obstructive sleep apnea. [2]

Long-term studies show the procedures cause significant and persistent loss of weight, recovery from diabetes, improvement in cardiovascular risk factors, and a reduction in mortality of 23% from 40%. [3]

However that could be misleading; a study in Veterans Affairs (VA) patients has found no survival benefit associated with bariatric surgery among older, severely obese people when compared with other more usual methods of weight control. [4]

Diabetes

Bariatric surgical intervention seems to be of special benefit to diabetics. A study from the Cleveland Clinic, published in 2013, helps to confirm this. Before surgery, only about half of patients had their blood sugar under control. After surgery, 80 percent of patients were well controlled.

The number of patients who required insulin therapy was reduced by half, and the number of patients requiring no medications rose 10-fold. In addition, patients significantly reduced their cardiovascular risk factors.

This somewhat striking effect lasted more than 5 years after surgery. Specifically, 24 percent of patients had complete remission of their diabetes with a blood sugar level of less than 6 percent without diabetes medications; another 26 percent had partial remission, while 34 percent of all patients had improved long-term diabetes control.

My comment on this is not to suggest bariatric surgery is the way to go but to point out that it is showing us the enormous benefit of making the effort to improve our eating and trim off all unnecessary pounds. Surgery is for seriously sick people and is not a short cut.

How It's Done

Most gastric bypass surgery is laparoscopic. The small incision from a laparoscope makes recovery time shorter. Most people stay in the hospital for two to three days, and resume normal activities in three to five weeks.

If the surgery must be "open" (requiring a large incision), healing time will take longer.

On average, people lose 61% of excess weight after gastric bypass surgery. Other surgeries such as gastric banding, result in about 47% of excess weight loss. 95% of cases report an improved quality of life.

Potential Problems After Weight Loss Surgery

Most people experience no serious problems after weight loss surgery, though 10% do have minor complications. Even that is enough to pause for thought, surely? Less than 5% experience serious (potentially life-threatening) complications.

Wound infections can happen up to three weeks after surgery. Symptoms include redness and warmth, pain, or thick drainage (pus) from the surgical wound. Wound infections require antibiotics and sometimes further surgery.

Constipation is common after weight loss surgery. Liquid cathartics like mineral oil can help. Avoid granular fiber (Metamucil or psyllium), which can cause obstructions.

Bleeding in the stool, which can appear as reddish or black stools, can be serious. Patients should let their doctor know about this immediately, or go to an emergency room.

Blood clots to the lungs, called pulmonary emboli, occur less than 1% of the time. They are the most common cause of death after weight loss surgery. Hey, there's no 1 in a 100 chance of death if you just eat less! Blood clots can usually be prevented with blood thinning drugs and frequent activity.

Leaks in the new connections made by the weight loss surgery are rare, but serious. They usually occur within five days of the surgery. Abdominal pain and feeling ill are common symptoms and either should warrant immediate attention.

Gallstones commonly occur with rapid weight loss. Up to 50% of people will develop gallstones after gastric bypass surgery; very painful but usually harmless. However, gallstones can cause nausea, vomiting, and abdominal pain, requiring more surgery. About 15% to 25% people require gallbladder removal after gastric bypass surgery.

So-called dumping syndrome (sudden fainting) occurs after eating high-sugar meals after weight loss surgery. Sodas or fruit juices are common culprits. The sugary food rushes through the stomach, whips up the blood sugar, followed by a compensatory state of hypoglycemia (low blood sugar) and that can cause nausea, vomiting, and weakness.

Bariatric surgery isn't for every temperament. Psychological screening is essential before bypass surgery but is sometimes ignored.[5]

Many weight loss surgery centers offer behavioral counseling programs. These can help people make the change to a healthier lifestyle before and after weight loss surgery.

Possible Complications

After weight-reduction surgery, the body may not absorb certain vitamins and minerals. Follow-up visits with your physician will determine which vitamin and mineral supplements are necessary after surgery.

Long-term complications of this malabsorption may include:

1. Anemia due to deficiency of iron or vitamin B12
2. Neurologic complications from vitamin B12 deficiency
3. Kidney stone disease due to changes in how the body absorbs calcium and oxalate
4. Possible bone disease due to mineral or vitamin D deficiency

5. Dehydration is a possible complication following weight-reduction surgery, as patients are no longer able to drink large quantities of liquid at one time (especially true in hot climates).
6. In the first three to six months after surgery, as the body reacts to rapid weight loss, the patient may experience one or more of the following changes (some changes are due to a slowing of the body's metabolism from weight loss and usually resolve with time):
    - Body aches
    - Feeling tired (flulike)
    - Feeling cold when others feel comfortable
    - Dry skin
    - Hair thinning and hair loss
    - Changes in mood
    - Relationship issues

Complications

TV celebrity Al Roker's embarrassing incontinence moment at the White House was awkward, but not uncommon. In fact, both fecal and urinary incontinence are common side effects of bariatric surgery that are little talked about. It may only be making an existing problem worse. According to a 2010 study, 55 percent of women and 31 percent of men with fecal incontinence felt their condition worsened after surgery.

Eating too quickly, taking big bites, not chewing enough or eating foods that are too dry can bring on nausea or vomiting in many people after weight-loss surgery, and too much sugary or greasy food can lead to diarrhea. More than a third of patients develop gallstones, masses of cholesterol that form in the gallbladder, after surgery.

About 20 percent of people who opt for weight-loss surgery require further procedures and as many as 30 percent deal with complications relating to malnutrition, like anemia or osteoporosis, since the intestines are absorbing fewer nutrients. So the side effects of these procedures can be dangerous and even life-threatening.

Mayo Clinic doctors have recognized and reported on a seemingly rare but serious complication following gastric bypass called post-bariatric surgery hypoglycemia. After a person eats, this condition can result in very low blood sugar levels that lead to severe neurologic symptoms, including visual disturbances, confusion and (rarely) seizures. Current treatment is to remove part of the pancreas.

Suicides

What's never talked about is that bariatric surgery patients seem to also be at greater risk of suicide. Calculated suicide rates among the patients can be more than five times higher than the rate in the general population, according to a review of nearly 17,000 operations performed from 1995 to 2004 in Pennsylvania. [6]

These suicides often take place after the initial 6-month close monitoring period and so the connection may not be made at all.

Conclusion and Recommendation

The idea of surgery as a quick fix is very far from the truth. Appetite and emotional cravings don't shrink just because stomach size does, and emotional issues need to be addressed. This is indicated by the fact that as many as 20% of patients gain back all their lost weight. When they aren't happy with the results, some patients, fall into a "rebound relationship with something else" reported ABC News, namely, alcohol, drugs or cigarettes.

Alexis Conason of the New York Obesity Nutrition Research Center, told ABC News that he found in his survey that surgery patients had a 50 percent increase in their frequency of substance abuse two years after their operations, particularly combined drug, tobacco and alcohol abuse. [7]

Bariatric surgery remains a violent and disturbing intervention, to help those who appear hopelessly addicted to food and will endure anything, to continue their reckless guzzling habits, without adequate exercise. It does not cure indolence or gluttony.

Of course surgeons will always be willing to perform this kind of operation, even though it is not actually healing as such. It's more a kind of rescue maybe.

However, there is an additional intriguing dimension to this story. Bypass surgery may alter our bowel flora in a favorable way...

Why Bypass Surgery Sometimes Works

In section 12 I pointed out the fact that our gut flora, or the microbiota as it's called, may be the main influence in the problem of obesity. With the right kind of intestinal flora, weight control is easy; but with the wrong microbes, staying slim can become a battle that's almost impossible to win.

New evidence suggests that this may be the main mechanism by which gastric bypass surgery succeeds. If so, surgery may become redundant, as we learn the trick of altering gut microbes. This is a surprise; most people would think intuitively that gastric bypass shrinks the stomach and rearranges the intestine enough to cause diminished food absorption.

But consider the new evidence and its implications:

It suggests that up to 20 percent of weight loss due to gastric bypass is brought about by altered gut flora, according to Dr. Lee M. Kaplan, director of the obesity, metabolism and nutrition institute at the Massachusetts General Hospital, and an author of a study published March 27th 2013, in *Science Translational Medicine*.

The researchers attempted to find out if microbial changes could account for some of the weight loss after gastric bypass. Earlier studies had shown that the microbiota of an obese person changed significantly after the surgery, becoming more like that of someone who was thin. But was the change from the surgery itself, or from the weight loss that followed the operation? And did the microbial change have any effects of its own?

To speed up the answers, Kaplan and his team used mice, which had been fed to the point of obesity. One batch had gastric bypass operations, and two other batches had "sham" operation (the animals' intestines were severed and sewn back together, to mimic any possible stress due to surgery).

Then the sham batch was further divided, some continuing to be fed on rich food, while the others were put on a weight-loss diet.[8]

The real bypass batch lost weight, obviously, but also their intestinal microbial populations quickly changed. In the sham batch, the microbiota did not change much, either in those continuing with a rich diet, or those on the weight-loss diet.

So far, nothing surprising.

But then the researchers transferred intestinal contents from each of the batches into other mice, which lacked their own intestinal bacteria. The animals that received fecal material from the bypass mice rapidly lost weight; stool from mice that had the sham operations had no effect.

The next step may be to take stool from people who have had gastric bypass and implant it into mice to see if causes them to lose weight. Then the same thing could be tried passing stool from person to person.

Anyone up for that? You have to want to really lose weight, I think![9]

PART 4. THE REST

SECTION 17. MIND STUFF

There is an extremely strong psychological relationship with food, which can make weight control difficult for many people. We like our food, it comforts us and we feel calm and relaxed after a good meal.

That's a parasympathetic effect, by the way: the opposite of sympathetic stimulation, which is what we get in the alarm phase (stress). Instead of wanting to rush away, in fight or flight mode, we just want to sit back and relax, watch a little TV... You know the feeling!

It's natural to become conditioned, in the Pavlovian sense, to want to eat. It satisfies many cravings and desires, above and beyond just the call for calories. It releases calming serotonin. We are rewarded for eating and therefore seek out this activity.

In caveman times, it was not easy to satisfy the craving for food: it took time, it was dangerous, hunting mammoths and dodging sabre-tooth tigers was pretty strenuous! But today, putting food on the table is so easy that we reward ourselves far too often.

In addition, as part of the modern age we are often actively encouraged to maintain a close emotional relationship with food. Think of all those TV ads which sweetly urge us to buy and consume more cookies "just like grandma used to make", or to unwind at the end of a busy day with our favorite brand of ice cream.

This is hypnotic manipulation, in the most wicked sense of the word.

Often the foods we are encouraged to desire are presented to us by extremely attractive men and women, cementing the subconscious, and often conscious, idea that eating as much as we like of such foods is a pleasure that comes with complete impunity – it may even make us happier and more gorgeous!

At best, such muddled thinking leads us down a path where ultimately when we are happy, we eat; when we are sad, we eat; when we are stressed, we eat; when we are celebrating, we eat; when we are angry, we eat; and so it goes on.

There is another bigger umbrella for this phenomenon. We are living in an age of anxiety, when everyone feels the fear of economic collapse, terrorism, ecological meltdown, water wars and worldwide pandemics. Our own little home environment is no longer a unit of safety and seclusion, as it once was. No matter how hard we work and how much we sequester away in the bank, we can never be truly safe. A world economic crisis could wipe out everything we have and put us back on the streets, fighting for food.

The responses to this constant "global stress", as I call it, are many and varied but the usual solutions are eating, drinking, sex and drugs (medical and street drugs). These tend to be the universal solutions for stress. The trouble is, you are not going to knock out these indulgent behaviors, if they truly are used as a solution. As we know, they are temporary, false solutions which, when used to excess, can cause even greater problems. To find a real solution you have to knock out the real problem and that isn't easy.

People Have Issues

In the meantime, we all know that the psychology of weight control is a major factor in keeping the pounds off. In a world which turns to eating for pleasure and comfort as well as survival, weight control is never going to be easy.

But we should also look at individual psychological issues. It is fair to say I think, speaking as an MD, that anyone who is 50 to 100 pounds or more overweight, has real problems inside their head. Just to allow your self-esteem to drop to the point where you couldn't care less how you look, where you are very uncomfortable waddling around, you don't look attractive, or when you have given up caring whether you live healthy or die young, is saying much deeper things about you than mere self-neglect. Many people who comfort eat or have over-eating disorders have experienced a trauma in childhood or adolescence.

Others may be translating their unresolved difficulties with home, school, work or love life into feelings of utter worthlessness. Very few people do not know that being overweight is bad for them at many levels, but in the most extreme cases over-eating can be viewed as a tortuously slow form of committing suicide.

The good news is that no one needs to continue to suffer by being overweight, with all the stresses, indignities, self-esteem challenges and health issues that this entails. I believe that anyone who genuinely wishes to help solve weight issues for people has to acknowledge that even a modest pamphlet on weight control would be incomplete without looking at the psychological aspects of dietary health.

So here we go...

Hypnotism

Probably the most popular and widely known technique in this regard is hypnotism. Many people hope that for them it will be a direct intervention into their psyche. Surely, if you can "adjust" a person's mindset to regard food less and not seek the indulgent solution to stress, then the weight will tend to come off naturally, without even resorting to a formula or program.

Some major figures who have worked with this, like Paul McKenna, claim good results. You may visit a specialist or purchase audio tracks that stand instead of an actual practitioner; meaning, his or her voice is on the audios. So for example, McKenna has his "I Can Make You Slim" set of audios, which have been popular.

A study in the *International Journal of Obesity* in 2005, which assessed 31 studies into complementary therapies, states that hypnosis had been proven in some cases to promote weight loss. This, however, does not tell us much more than what we already know from friends and anecdotes. It seems probable that hypnotherapy may go some way to reinforce positive dietary habits, the will to exercise and the will-power to stop snacking, etc.

However, research also states that it is not a 'one size fits all' solution, or necessarily effective for those who have more than a little weight to lose. Hypnosis works for some; indeed I can say it's disappointing that it doesn't work for everybody: they say some people are hypnotizable and some are not.

A few studies have evaluated the use of weight-loss hypnosis. Most studies showed only slight weight loss, with an average loss of about 6 pounds (2.7 kilograms). But the quality of some of these studies has been questioned, making it hard to determine the true effectiveness of weight-loss hypnosis.

Slimming is usually best achieved with diet and exercise. If you've tried diet and exercise but are still struggling to meet your weight-loss goal, talk to your health care provider about other options or lifestyle changes that you can make. Don't rely on weight-loss hypnosis alone because it's unlikely to lead to significant weight loss. [1]

My good friend Elaine Kissel PhD, a professional and skilled hypnotherapist, disagrees that some people cannot be hypnotized and thinks failures are down to the lack of ability in individual practitioners. She has this to say:

"Hypnosis is a powerful tool. It serves the therapist and client in myriad ways. It can be employed to glean insights into the often deep-rooted and complex issues that motivate excess eating and weight and resolve them at the root level; it can then be used to facilitate the development of healthy eating patterns. Teaching the client healthy coping strategies, and the use of self-hypnosis as a means of supporting the therapeutic process is vital to success. Hypnosis is in and of itself therapeutic, enabling natural relaxation and stress relief."

Health Coaching

Weight loss which is supported by health coaching can be extremely effective. Health coaching is essentially the holistic support and advice from one individual to another to motivate a positive change. The leading modern health coaches use techniques which inspire their clients to make conscious changes to the way they think and feel to enjoy a better outcome.

A health or wellness coach may be one of the functions of a personal trainer, who will not only oversee an exercise regime, some will also look at emotional, psychological, mental and dietary changes for the better.

Health coaching may include instances of motivational interviewing. Originally used to help people with alcohol problems, it is a mode of coaching where the coach targets the take-it-or-leave-it attitude towards change (which is really fear) that plagues so many people who are trying to make an important improvement in their life, such as losing weight.

Motivational interviewing is a specific skill and more targeted than general counseling. When it comes to promoting weight loss, the health coach will work closely with their client to ask probing questions such as:

- How do you feel about losing weight?
- What do you think life will be like after you lose weight?
- Will weight loss change you as a person?
- What scares you about this change?
- Are there downsides to losing weight?
- What do you feel are the main barriers to losing weight?

By discussing directly relevant hopes and fears in detail, examining the big, scary idea of change and addressing it once and for all, health coaches can help their clients guide themselves towards better futures. If you have ever loved the truth of the great movie quotes about being afraid of happiness, or fear of failure, then you will understand the potential power that a health coach can have.

In the Oscar-winning movie *Little Miss Sunshine*, Grandpa says:

"Losers are people who are so afraid of not winning, they don't even try."

So many people who want to get rid of their excess weight feel exactly this way. A great health coach can teach them that deep down, they know that trying is nothing to be scared of and it is the only way to be healthy and happy.

Targeted Psychotherapy

A staggering 43 percent of those who have weight issues attribute the majority of their problems to emotional causes. Some people have experienced issues in the past, which they tried to solve by eating and they are now literally carrying the problems around with them as excess fat.

In such cases it makes sense to get to the root of the problem. Over 70 percent of psychologists who specialize in helping people with weight issues approach the problem in three different ways:

1. Cognitive Therapy

This is a treatment where people are helped to identify and finally address the negative emotions or thoughts which have led to the behaviors that are causing them problems by reasoning things through. In other words, if someone overeats because they dislike themselves for some reason—often without realizing it—that issue can be addressed.

To my mind this works in the same way as ensuring the foundations of a house are stable. No one would try to improve the appearance of the bedrooms if the foundations were crumbling, would they? If someone wants to become a healthy weight and stay that way, it is essential that they look after their mental foundations.

2. Finding Practical Solutions

A psychologist will look into ways of finding alternative solutions to the problems that we face on a daily basis. Rather than try to solve them by eating food, we can empower ourselves by dealing with challenges head-on, using the techniques offered. Some of those may include goal-setting, keeping a food/mood diary and motivational strategies, including non-food incentives.

3. Mindfulness

This is essentially a way in which you can live in and be aware of each moment without constant self-criticism and blame. It is allied to the state one achieves with meditation and can also be a positive part of Neuro-Linguistic Programming (NLP); see below. But mindfulness also stands alone as a way of training your mind to be present and therefore more positive. Practiced regularly as part of therapy it can be a very useful tool.

No one should enter lightly into a course of therapy, but if you know, or simply suspect, that there are deeper issues which are causing you to eat too much or which may be stopping you from being the healthy person that you want to be, it is a great idea to seek help for those issues. Don't ever neglect your mental foundations if you want your body, or 'house', to be the best home for a positive spirit.

Meditation

Meditation has long been familiar to the West as an ancient practice which can be used for stress relief, or to calm what Meg Ryan once described in an interview as a having a "chatty mind". The star of *When Harry Met Sally* is an advocate of meditation, saying:

"By simply refocusing our awareness, we reshape our experience."

This reassuring truth can also be applied to day-to-day battles with food and weight. Meditation is increasingly being studied as a means by which we can prevent weight gain and obesity, or encourage weight loss and better all-round health.

Research has shown that the effects on eating patterns after using meditation can be profound and beneficial. The relaxing effect may stop food from being misused to salve emotions, such as in the case of binge eating. However, one even more important effect may be the new awareness that the person may experience, a pure awareness about eating that is the opposite of the swinging back and forth of guilt, despair and blame versus the dieter's hope; self-hatred and self-disgust versus pride in 'being good for a change'. These are extreme qualities which meditation can remove and so help someone finally "see things as they really are."

This aspect is vital, since laboratory research into the regulation of eating clearly demonstrates that people who have issues relating to weight and eating tend to be far less aware of when they are genuinely hungry as opposed to just being bored, or experiencing an emotional trigger or simply having a bit of healthy appetite. They are also less aware of feeling full, or of when their body has had enough. It is easy to see why practicing self-awareness could help in such cases.

Which brings us back to where we began this chapter—the crucial understanding that thoughts and emotions frequently drive us to over-indulge in food. It makes sense that being aware of an unhealthy behavior at the level of the initial thought or impulse could help us alter that behavior.

In fact by getting the patient to simply be aware of the precise moment of eating, greater self-control became much easier.

Neuro-Linguistic Programming (NLP)

Connirae Andreas PhD, an internationally known trainer and researcher in NLP, coauthor of the marvelous book *Heart Of The Mind*, gives a very simple technique, which I have tried, taught others, and found to be extremely valuable.

She calls it the Naturally-Slender Eating Strategy! We all do different things in our minds, when we think about work, love, pleasure and eating. These structured sequences of thought are what NLP practitioners call "mind strategies". Connirae points out that people who are slim, eat well and stay healthy must be doing something different than the rest of us when they think about food. Something that helps them control their eating desires.

Since she is a naturally slim person, Connirae asked herself "What goes on in my mind when I start to think about food?" Her answer went something like this:

1. I check how my stomach feels now.
2. I ask myself "What would feel good in my stomach?"
3. I imagine a portion of food: a sandwich, a bowl of soup, etc.
4. I visualize eating this food and get the feeling of how this amount of food will feel in my stomach over time, if I eat it now and it stays in my system for some hours to come.
5. If I like this feeling better than the feeling of not eating at all, I keep this food item as a possibility.
6. She repeats this for several food options and then, when she has enough choices, she finally picks the one that she knows will feel best over time.
7. She feels good after eating that food because she spent a lot of thought making sure she would!

That's a "no guilt" strategy, as you can readily see. Unfortunately, for most obese people, their mental strategy goes rather like this:

1. I think about food.
2. I realize I feel hungry.
3. I like pizza pie.
4. I'll eat pizza pie, probably a second helping because I really LIKE pizza pie.
5. I give no thought for how this will make me feel over time.
6. I eat the food and maybe another helping.
7. About half an hour after eating, I start to feel yuck in my stomach.
8. I start wishing I hadn't eaten that.
9. Soon I start thinking about food all over again and fall into the same dumb strategy, even though I know it doesn't work.

Contrast this last with Connirae's own food strategy and you'll soon realize why she's slim and you are maybe not!

Can Stress Make You Gain Weight?

You bet it can. But not just because, when we are stressed, we reach for comfort foods. It's more complicated than that.

Increasingly, modern life can trigger a stress response from us. It could be after a hard day at work, not being able to pay a bill, or even being faced with the possibility of assault. Whether it is a fight-or-flight moment, or sustained pressure, the biochemical result is that we go into survival mode.

This sounds helpful and it can be to an organism under threat, but not to someone who wants to lose weight. Why? When we are stressed, out metabolism slows down, we store fuel and the system becomes loaded with cortisol as well as other important hormones. These combine to increase the likelihood of putting on abdominal fat.

Of course it's true that when stressed we often reach for 'comfort' foods more readily. We go for high carb foods at such time because these increase serotonin in the brain, which makes us feel better for a while. Whilst stressed, we may also sleep less soundly, which as I have previously mentioned, can have a negative impact on our food choices. Naturally, food never solves the problems causing the stress and can add to it by ultimately making you even more unhappy about your weight. The key is to fix the root of the problem rather than bingeing on unhealthy foods.

Earlier in this book (section 11), we looked at the impact that cortisol, the "stress hormone" can have on the body. It is important to understand, so it is worth going over the key aspects again here.

Cortisol, which is secreted by the adrenal glands, is essential and has many roles to play within the body. Normally, cortisol levels are high in the morning and low later in the day, when we naturally switch to parasympathetic mode (relaxed). Cortisol is critical for regulating blood pressure and providing energy, stimulates the metabolism of fat and carbohydrate to rapidly give energy, and prompts insulin release and helps with the maintenance of blood sugar levels. All of these actions can lead to an increase in appetite.

When we are stressed, over active, we produce excessive cortisol and the diurnal pattern where cortisol is high in the morning and low at night, is disrupted. This disruption may lead to weight gain, which may moreover be in the worst area: the belly. As we know, toxic belly fat increases the likelihood of heart attack and stroke.

It is therefore well worth taking steps to reduce all this fat-inducing stress as much as possible.

Fix Chronic Stress By Tuning It Out

Maximize your weight-loss chances by doing what you can to minimize stress. Try these stress-busting ideas:

Yoga and Tai Ch'i. In the latter half of the twentieth century, a number of Asian practices suddenly appeared in the West. Although these were unfamiliar, it seems that we quickly took them to heart and began practicing them. Yoga has many forms, which we do not need to detail here. Let's just say: find one you like. Tai Ch'i is similar, in harnessing natural body "energies", but is more relaxing, less awkward, and therefore can be practiced by people who are carrying too much body weight.

In the end, it comes down to what you can find in your locality and what feels right for you.

Brain Entrainment. It's all about brainwaves! You can do this on a practiced basis, using methods such as Silva mind control. It's really just dropping your mind activity into a relaxed, semi-inward state, we call alpha. Meditation and "mindfulness" can do it too. These are not easy to adopt but can be learned by anyone with enough determination.

There are also electronic devices to help you. You have probably heard about binaural beats and brain entrainment devices. But today there is much more technology available than just binaurals.

State-of-the-art equipment will enable you to bring to bear four different relaxing modalities, to be sure your brain gets the calming message!

Binaural beats have been around since Dr. Gerald Oster of the Mt. Sinai Medical Center, published his ground-breaking paper entitled "Auditory Beats in the Brain" in the October 1973 issue of *Scientific American.*

But the story isn't limited to binaural beats. Even more powerful as a means of brain entrainment is photic driving or flicker following (flashing lights). These were described by Walter Grey as early as the 1940s.

Couple these together with soothing music (slow Baroque style is said to be best) and a gentle, healing voice that gives you guiding thoughts towards escaping from everyday stress, using mind imagery and you have what I call multi-media sensory stimulation or MMSS.

There are two outstanding devices of this nature. One, The Kasina, you can find on my websites at: www.alternative-doctor.com/getthekasina/

The other is the Brain Tap, developed by Patrick Porter. This device has its own "app", which may highly appeal to smartphone geeks.

Learn more here: http://braintaptechnology.com/bt/drscott-mumby or get a free trial here: http://braintapstore.com/freetrial/drscott-mumby

Exercise. The feeling of healthy tiredness and well-being after exercise is great. Whether you run, dance or do yoga, movement makes you feel good and helps to relieve stress; even taking a walk in the fresh air can blow away the day's stress. Talking of which...sex. It's worth mentioning that love-making with the consenting adult of your choice is not just wonderful on a romantic level, it is also one of Nature's very best de-stressors

After the sexual act, we find ourselves in the parasympathetic state. This is the eat, relax, sleep mode; we find ourselves like that after eating. Well, if weight is a problem, sex is a better way to get there than eating... Just saying!

For longer lasting solutions to hidden and deeper levels of hurt and insecurity, I highly commend my own technique of piloting. It's a way of getting to the unaddressed origins of unpleasant and unwanted emotional states, the times when we were in sympathetic overload: in other words, fight or flight mode. This is something that any of us can learn to do, to help Self and even to help others after a little practice.

You can learn more by reading my book "Punk Psychology®". It's a joke label but does emphasize the fact that it is very different, edgy and way off the mainstream axis. Learn more at:

www.punkpsychology.us

PART 4. THE REST

SECTION 18. LONG-TERM MAINTENANCE

What is very depressing, and nobody wants to happen, is to work hard and take the weight off, only to put it all back on again.

But you can beat the trend which, after all, only comes from short-term thinking: "I'll lose the weight and then...." Most people are very silly and make all the necessary effort, but look forward, when it's over, to getting back to their favorite ice cream, candies or pizzas.

Get rid of this thinking. Set yourself up on a 5-year plan, not a 5-week spurt. Five years is a long time but you don't have to be tough on yourself the whole time. The first few weeks or months are about losing the weight; from then on it's about keeping the weight off, which is much easier.

But keeping it off has to be part of the plan!

The US National Weight Control Registry (NWCR) is currently tracking over 10,000 individuals who have lost significant amounts of weight (at least 30 lbs. or 13.6 kilos) and kept it off for a significant period of time, so these are people you need to listen to.

Detailed questionnaires and annual follow-up surveys are used to examine the behavioral and psychological characteristics of successful weight loss individuals, as well as the strategies they use for maintaining their weight loss.

For example, members report engaging in high levels of physical activity (approximately one hour per day); eating a low-calorie, low-fat diet (probably a hangover from the days when this was fashionable); eating breakfast regularly; self-monitoring weight; and maintaining a consistent eating pattern across weekdays and weekends.

Obviously, weight loss maintenance may get easier over time; after individuals have successfully maintained their weight loss for 2-5 years, the chance of longer-term success greatly increases. [1]

What Have We Learned?

Figures from the registry tell an interesting story:

- 80% of persons in the registry are women and 20% are men.
- The "average" woman is 45 years of age and currently weighs 145 lbs, while the "average" man is 49 years of age and currently weighs 190 lbs.
- Registry members have lost an average of 66 lbs. and kept it off for 5.5 years.

These averages, however, hide a lot of diversity:

- Weight losses have ranged from 30 to 300 lbs.
- Duration of successful weight loss has ranged from 1 year to 66 years!
- Some have lost the weight rapidly, while others have lost weight very slowly, over as many as 14 years.

We can also take a look at how the weight loss was accomplished:

- 45% of registry participants lost the weight on their own and the other 55% lost weight with the help of some type of program.
- 98% of registry participants report that they modified their food intake in some way to lose weight.
- 94% increased their physical activity, with the most frequently reported form of activity being walking.

There is variety in how NWCR members keep the weight off. Most report continuing to maintain a low calorie, low fat diet and doing high levels of activity.

- 78% eat breakfast every day.
- 75% weigh themselves at least once a week.
- 62% watch less than 10 hours of TV per week.
- 90% exercise, on average, about 1 hour per day.

Eating paleo most of the time is a lot easier than all that exercise, I can tell you that.

Successful Strategies

Successful long-term strategies can be summed up then, as follows:

Get Active and Stay Active. As I said earlier, exercise isn't the best way to lose weight but it's a very important way to keep the weight off!

There are many other benefits to an active life, other than just weight control; for example, helping blood fats, reducing blood pressure, reducing stress, improving mood and well-being, and strengthening the heart.

Find something you love and dedicate yourself to it, whether it's dancing, walking, biking, or playing sports.

Gym advisories often talk about cardio exercises, as if they helped with weight. Cardio is worthless for weight loss. It's interval training (short bursts of intense activity) that scores highest. This is true aerobic exercise, not the ersatz version.

Try to get out of breath at least once a day.

Keep A Journal.

Multiple studies show that people who keep a journal to track the foods they eat lose more weight and keep it off for the long haul. In fact, the NWCR has found that logging foods is one way successful losers stay on track well after they've lost the intended weight. In another study published in the *American Journal of Preventive Medicine*, those who used a food diary while dieting lost twice as much weight as those who didn't.

Drink Water - Sensibly

Do NOT drink 6 – 8 glasses a day: for many people that's way too much and will increase blood pressure. Do not fall for the corny myth that all water is good. You can have too much of a good thing.

The point here is to drink water before food and drink; it will help to kill your appetite. If you live in a hot climate, drink more; if not, regulate your intake sensibly.

Join A Buddy Or Support Group

Again, the NWCR tells us that those who lost weight successfully and continued going to bi-monthly support group meetings for a year maintained their weight. Those who didn't go to support meetings regained almost half of the weight they lost.

The important point, obviously, is to be accountable to some other person or group. Your life partner or spouse might be the right person for that; maybe not!

Don't Worry, Be Happy!

Stress and low mood are serious enemies of weight control. Whatever your life issues may be, get them fixed up. Nobody likes being unhappy anyway, by definition.

Weight control is actually a whole-life issue and needs approaching accordingly, not just as an add-on or afterthought.

Remember how you were.

Remember my wife Vivien's tip of keeping a photo of yourself around, showing yourself as you were at your best. Let it remind and inspire you to more effort and less indulgence.

Keeping a photo of your past self in your purse or wallet also comes in handy when you're tempted to skip a scheduled workout or tempted to make an unhealthy option while dining out.

Keep Weighing Yourself.

For at least the first 5 years of your new self, keep a check. Don't let things slip. Nothing is as difficult to control as the slow, insidious, pound by pound increase in fat that takes place if you are not monitoring your health and weight. The only way to spot the slide is to look for it! Check at least weekly.

About three-quarters of all successful long-term weight-loss maintainers from the NWCR report that they weigh themselves weekly to keep the extra pounds at bay.

But also the fit of your clothes is a good monitor. If those special jeans start to get tight again, look out! Back to the scales, back to your successful actions and re-assert your resolve to continue looking great... forever!

It only remains for me to wish you the very best of endeavors!

APPENDIX

Top 10 FREE Weight Loss Phone Apps

A survey reported by Health.com found 35% of us use an app before even getting out of bed in the morning.

At least one study suggests it may be a good idea to use a smartphone app to coach people as they try to shed extra pounds. This kind of gadget interactivity, which is so popular today (known as applications or apps for short), may make a standard weight-loss program more effective.

That's a relief because calorie-counting apps for smart phones have literally exploded in numbers.

But here's a reality check: it does need to be a part of a comprehensive and effective weight loss program.

Researchers at Northwestern University studied about 70 overweight men. Their average age was 58, so they weren't exactly born with smartphones in their hands.

Some of the men were asked to log their eating and activity using old-fashioned pen and pad; these were the controls. Others were given a mobile app, and their behaviors were monitored by a coach who provided short, telephone-based check-in sessions periodically during the study. In addition, all of the participants were offered group classes in nutrition and behavior change.

The smartphone app definitely helped. Those who used one and also attended 80 percent of the health education classes lost 15 lbs. more than the controls and were able to keep it off for at least a year, the researchers reported.

The report was published online Dec. 10 2012 in the *Archives of Internal Medicine.*

For the study, 69 overweight and obese patients, average age about 58, were randomly assigned to a standard weight-loss program or a weight-loss program with smartphone prompting. The programs lasted one year. The volunteers were weighed at three, six, nine and 12 months.

Patients who were coached using smartphones lost more than those in the standard weight-loss program, the findings showed. In addition, about one-third of those in the smartphone program lost at least 5 percent of their body weight when they were only three months into the program, while those in the other group lost nothing during that time period.

So if nothing else, a smart phone weight loss app watching over you is a great way to get started in earnest.

Interestingly, neither the phone app alone nor the group weight-loss classes were effective for the average patient. It was the *combination* of technology and health education which worked effectively.

So, should you get one? The answer lies partly in your temperament. If you can identify yourself as an individual who needs extra motivation and discipline, something to keep you accountable and you like playing with your smartphone or tablet environment... then yes!

Not being a smartphone geek myself, I have relied on the opinions of others to get you started. The majority of these top weight loss and/or exercise monitoring apps are the recommendation of Jennifer Cohen (shared 8/21/2012 @ 6:44 pm). She posted them on the Forbes website. They are all available as free downloads on most popular Smart Phone platforms.

1. Lose It!

This free app lets you look up food to track calories and track your exercise in the same app. Just input your current weight and your goal weight, and **Lose It!** will give you a fairly accurate estimate of how many calories to eat per day, and how long it should take to reach that goal. There's even an online support community you can join where people like you can encourage and hold each other accountable. You can also scan the barcodes of almost any item and automatically pull calorie and nutritional info from a huge online database of product items.

Free: Apple, Android

2. Fooducate

Fooducate helps you spot those tricky non-health foods quickly by cutting your research time in half. Simply scan the barcode and Fooducate will give you a rating for the food scanned based on calorie counts per serving, processing techniques and amount of excess sugar.

On test, it steered the user away from a honey wheat bread (a mere C+, because of refined flour) and toward an equally tasty 100% whole-wheat loaf (A-). That's unfortunate and shows ignorance of the effects of wheat. If you don't tolerate wheat very well (most people don't) then whole-wheat is a double whammy—very concentrated and impactful.

Free: Apple, Android

3. Locavore

(Like carnivore!) Locavore tells you what's in season, how old the food item is likely to be and how many days you have left to enjoy it's nutritional value and flavor. It can also use your phone's GPS to find the closest places to buy locally grown, in-season produce. Many people have never tasted really fresh vegetables and when they do... many find they like it more than they knew. Buy in season, fresh and local whenever you can and you'll turn on to your 5-a-day.

Free: Apple, Android

4. Nike Training Club

This app is a free personal trainer in your pocket. It has 30-45 minute timed workouts for cardio, toning and strength, videos for each move and a voiceover talking you though the workout, and it pulls music from your own playlists to keep you motivated. Just choose a workout based on the time you have and the results you want, and press play. You can also turn on autoshare, holding yourself accountable to all of your Facebook friends. One of the most unique parts of this app is the reward features, which make working out into a game. The step-by-step videos and integration with your own music library make this a great personal workout app.

Free: Apple

5. Endomondo

If you're a runner, biker or walker, this app will track your route via Google Maps, tracking your work-out history to compare later. You can also create an account and get motivated by your friends every time you break a mile. You can even upgrade the app to work with special Polar heart rate monitors.

Free: Apple, Android, Blackberry

6. My Fitness Pal

My Fitness Pal takes your weight, height, goal weight and lifestyle into account before giving its recommendations. It breaks up your big goal into a smaller goal, one month away, which makes the milestones seem friendlier. You can also access calorie counts and nutritional information from local restaurants, taking the guesswork out of eating out. You can also access your calorie count online from any computer, and get some extra encouragement by sharing your progress with friends.

Free: Apple, Android

7. Eat This, Not That! The Game

Jennifer Cohen is more reserved about this one. Is it a good idea to choose one bad fast food over another (chili dogs over cheeseburgers? Really?) It could possibly help some people who are hopelessly addicted to the occasional burger or hot dog. There could also be situations (I've found myself in them sometimes) where there is no good choice and it would be nice to know you chose the best you could. It works as a game and like all games, you can find yourself using up time you cannot really spare.

Free: Apple, Android

Now Some Paid Apps

The website health.com suggests some more apps which are NOT free:

8. Meal Snap

This app analyzes a pic of your plate, then gives you a ballpark calorie range. Testers tried it on a steak, rice, and roasted asparagus plate at the local steakhouse, which clocked in at between 329 and 434 calories (a nicely modest splurge).

($0.99; Apple devices)

9. The Carb Lover's Diet

Health.com's own app not only offers loads of tasty recipes for waistline-conscious carboholics, but also a weight-loss planner to track carbs and calories.

Where else can you lose weight eating coconut French toast?

(free, but with $4.99 upgrade; go to iTunes; for iPhone, iPod Touch, iPad)

10. Shake a Snack

Give your device a jiggle, and a virtual slot machine rings up a three-ingredient snack for 100 to 300 calories.

Testers for Health.com scored a totally yummy 170-calorie Greek yogurt–pumpkin–graham cracker creation.

($0.99; shakeasnack.com; for iPhone, iPod Touch, iPad)

If you are the kind of person who would enjoy one of these apps, the chances are you know how to surf the web and will no doubt find more examples for yourself!

REFERENCES

SECTION 1

1 Eur Heart J (2012) 33 (8): 998-1006

2 *British Journal Of Sports Medicine*, 8 Sep 2016. http://dx.doi.org/10.1136/bjsports-2016-096194

3 *University of Exeter, news release, Dec. 7, 2011*

4 *J Obes*. 2011;2011. pii: 297315. doi: 10.1155/2011/297315. Epub 2010 Aug 10

5 Segerstrom SC, Miller GE. Psychological stress and the human immune system: a meta-analytic study of 30 years of inquiry. *Psychol Bull*. 2004;130(4):601–30

SECTION 2

1 *Am J Clin Nutr* June 2004 vol. 79 no. 6 946-961

2 Sept. 4, 2009, *British Medical Journal*

3 *J Am Diet Assoc*. 1994 Aug;94(8):855-8

4 Kong, A. Journal of the Academy of Nutrition and Dietetics, July 13, 2012

5 SOURCE: Annual meeting of the Society for the Study of Ingestive Behavior, Zurich, July 10-14, 2012

SECTION 3

1 Dr. Mercola: http://articles.mercola.com/sites/articles/archive/2009/02/10/new-study-of-splenda-reveals-shocking-information-about-potential-harmful-effects.aspx

2 Effects of dietary glycemic index on brain regions related to reward and craving in men 1,2,3,4. *The American Journal of Clinical Nutrition*, June 26, 2013

3 Morrison JF, Shehab S, Sheen R, Dhanasekaran S, Shaffiullah M, Mensah- Brown E; "Sensory And Autonomic Nerve Changes In The Msg-Treated Rat : A Model Of Type II Diabetes"; UAE University

4 *American Journal of Clinical Nutrition*, June 2011

5 http://www.foodnavigator.com/Science/Phosphate-in-food-is-health-risk-that-should-be-labelled-claim-researchers

6 de Vendômois JS, Roullier F, Cellier D, Séralini GE. A Comparison of the Effects of Three GM Corn Varieties on Mammalian Health. Int J Biol Sci 2009; 5(7):706-726. doi:10.7150/ijbs.5.706.

7 Judy A. Carman, Howard R. Vlieger, Larry J. Ver Steeg, Verlyn E. Sneller, Garth W. Robinson, Catherine A. Clinch-Jones, Julie I. Haynes, John W. Edwards (2013). A long-term toxicology study on pigs fed a combined genetically modified (GM) soy and GM maize diet. *Journal of Organic Systems* 8 (1): 38-54. Open access full text: http://www.organic-systems.org/journal/81/8106.pdf

8 Gilles-Eric Séralini et al., Long term toxicity of a Roundup herbicide and a Roundup-tolerant genetically modified maize; *Food and Chemical Toxicology* 50 (2012) 4221–4231... if you can find it. It was withdrawn under pressure

9 http://GMseralini.org/ten-things-you-need-to-know-about-the-seralini-study/ accessed Oct 16 2013, 7.00 am BST

10 http://www.webmd.com/food-recipes/features/are-biotech-foods-safe-to-eat, accessed Sep 16, 2013, 9.00 am BST.

SECTION 4

1 Cummings DE, Weigle DS, Frayo RS, Breen PA, Ma MK, Dellinger EP, Purnell JQ (May 2002). "Plasma ghrelin levels after diet-induced weight loss or gastric bypass surgery". N. Engl. J. Med. 346 (21): 1623–30.

2 http://en.wikipedia.org/wiki/Ghrelin

3 Díez JJ, Iglesias P (March 2003). "The role of the novel adipocyte-derived hormone adiponectin in human disease". Eur. J. Endocrinol. 148 (3): 293–300. As cited by Wikipedia http://en.wikipedia.org/wiki/Adiponectin

4 Expert Rev Anti Infect Ther. 2012;10(5):521-524

5 "Virus Is Linked To Weight Problems In Humans" by Marilynn Marchione, Milwaukee Journal Sentinel (from Seattle Post-Intelligencer on Tuesday Morning, April 8, 1997)

6 Anderson, RA. "Effects of chromium on body composition and weight loss." *Nutri Rev.* 1998 Sep; 56-(9): 266-70

7 Kaats GR, et al. "The effects of chromium picolinate supplementation on body composition." *Current Therapeutic Research.* Feb 1996

8 Schroeder, H.A. (1968). The role of chromium in mammalian nutrition. *American Journal of Clinical Nutrition*, 21, 230-244

1 *The Lancet*, Volume 373, Issue 9669, Pages 1083 - 1096, 28 March 2009

2 Weisberg SP, McCann D, Desai M, Rosenbaum M, Leibel RL, Ferrante AW Jr. Obesity is associated with macrophage accumulation in adipose tissue. J Clin Invest. 2003; 112: 1796–1808

SECTION 7

1 Nanji AA, Freeman JB. Relationship between body weight and total leukocyte count in morbid obesity. Am J Clin Pathol. 1985; 84: 346–347

2 Cottam DR, Mattar SG, Barinas-Mitchell E, Eid G, Kuller L, Kelley DE, Schauer PR. The chronic inflammatory hypothesis for the morbidity associated with morbid obesity: implications and effects of weight loss. Obes Surg. 2004; 14: 589–600

3 Fontana L, Eagon JC, Trujillo ME, Scherer PE, Klein S. Visceral fat adipokine secretion is associated with systemic inflammation in obese humans. Diabetes, published online Feb. 7, 2007

4 World J Hepatol. 2015 Jun 18; 7(11): 1450–1459

5 Klein, S. New England Journal of Medicine, June 17, 2004; vol 350: pp 2549-2557

6 Yang ZH, Miyahara H, Hatanaka A. Chronic administration of palmitoleic acid reduces insulin resistance and hepatic lipid accumulation in KK-Ay Mice with genetic type 2 diabetes. Lipids Health Dis. 2011;10:120

7 Bernstein AM, Roizen MF, Martinez L. Purified palmitoleic acid for the reduction of high-sensitivity C-reactive protein and serum lipids: a double-blinded, randomized, placebo controlled study. J Clin Lipidol. 2014;8(6):612-7

8 Mozaffarian D, Cao H, King IB, et al. Circulating palmitoleic acid and risk of metabolic abnormalities and new-onset diabetes. Am J Clin Nutr. 2010;92(6):1350-8

9 Lancet. 2011 Feb 12;377(9765):557-67

10 http://www.thedailybeast.com/newsweek/2009/09/10/born-to-be-big.html

11 *Washington Post*, Monday, March 12, 2007, By Elizabeth Grossman. Accessed Aug 7th, 2013, 5.50 pm. BST

SECTION 8

1 Brandon Gaille website: https://brandongaille.com/27-awesome-sugar-consumption-statistics/

2 Chiarelli F, Marcovecchio ML. Insulin resistance and obesity in childhood. *Eur J Endocrinol* 2008; 159(Suppl 1):S67–S74

3 BMJ 1995;311:1401

4 Da Villa G, Ianiro G, Mangiola F, et al. White mulberry supplementation as adjuvant treatment of obesity. J Biol Regul Homeost Agents. 2014 Jan-Mar;28(1):141-5

SECTION 9

1 Venga R, Good M, Howard P, and Vacek J, Role Of Vitamin D In Cardiovascular Health, *American J Cardiology*, 2010; 106; 798-805

2 see Death by Calcium: Proof of the Toxic Effects of Dairy and Calcium Supplements by Thomas E. Levy MD, JD. 2013

3 *Mol Nutr Food Res.* 2011 Jan;55(1):136-49

4 *Arch Pediatr Adolesc Med.* 2010 Apr;164(4):328-33

5 Obesity (Silver Spring) 19: 212–215

6 J Nutr Biochem. 2008 Dec;19(12):840-7

7 Cutting edge: progesterone directly upregulates vitamin d receptor gene expression for efficient regulation of T cells by calcitriol. J Immunol. 2015 Feb 1;194(3):883-6. doi: 10.4049/jimmunol.1401923. Epub 2014 Dec 29

8 Fahey JW, Holtzclaw WD, Wehage SL, Wade KL, Stephenson KK, Talalay P (2015) Sulforaphane Bioavailability from Glucoraphanin-Rich Broccoli: Control by Active Endogenous Myrosinase. PLoS ONE 10(11): e0140963. doi:10.1371/journal.pone.0140963

9 Fahey JW, Holtzclaw WD, Wehage SL, Wade KL, Stephenson KK, Talalay P (2015) Sulforaphane Bioavailability from Glucoraphanin-Rich Broccoli: Control by Active Endogenous Myrosinase. PLoS ONE 10(11): e0140963. doi:10.1371/journal.pone.0140963

10 "British Journal of Nutrition"; Dissociation of the Glycaemic and Insulinaemic Responses to Whole and Skimmed Milk; Garrett Hoyt, et al.; 2005

SECTION 10

1 *Diabetes Obes Metab.* 2010 Jan;12(1):72-81. doi: 10.1111/j.1463-1326.2009.01132.x. Epub 2009 Oct 13

2 Oben JE, et al. Irvingia gabonensis significantly reduces body weight and improves metabolic parameters in overweight humans. *Lipids in Health and Disease.* 2009, 8:7

3 Reuters, "Exotic Fruit Extract May Shed Pounds, Lower Cholesterol," March 24, 2009. FOXNews.com

4 Grossman, A. "Turmeric Extract Suppresses Fat Tissue Growth in Rodent Models," Tufts University, news.tufts.edu May 18, 2009

5 For example: Anand P, Sundaram C, Jhurani S, Kunnumakkara AB, Aggarwal BB.Curcumin and cancer: an "old-age" disease with an "age-old" solution. *Cancer Lett.* 2008 Aug 18;267(1):133-64

6 *Adv Exp Med Biol.* 2007;595:1-75

7 Kuriyan R, et al. Effect of Caralluma fimbriata extract on appetite. *Appetite.* 2007 May;48(3):338-44

8 http://www.webmd.com/vitamins-supplements/ingredientmono-1160-CARALLUMA.aspx?activeIngredientId=1160&activeIngredientName=CARALLUMA

9 This finding was backed up by another study, conducted by MacLean DB, Luo LG. "Increased ATP content/production in the hypothalamus may be a signal for energy-sensing of satiety: studies of the anorectic mechanism of a plant steroidal glycoside." *Brain Res.* 2004 Sep 10;1020(1-2):1-11

10 see also: van Heerden FR, Marthinus Horak R, Maharaj VJ, Vleggaar R, Senabe JV, Gunning PJ. An appetite suppressant from Hoodia species. *Phytochemistry.* 2007 Oct;68(20):2545-53. Epub 2007 Jul 2

11 http://en.wikipedia.org/wiki/Nelumbo_nucifera

12 *Am. J. Bot.* February 2002 vol. 89 no. 2 236-247

13 Ono Y, et al. Anti-obesity effect of Nelumbo nucifera leaves extract in mice and rats. *J Ethnopharmacol.* 2006 Jun 30;106(2):238-44

14 www.sensa.com retrieved 7/12/2013 at 9.30 am BST

15 "Xenical Pharmacology, Pharmacokinetics, Studies, Metabolism". http://www.rxlist.com/xenical-drug/clinical-pharmacology.htm Retrieved 2013- 07-10.

16 Padwal R, Li SK, Lau DC (2004). "Long-term pharmacotherapy for obesity and overweight". In Padwal, Raj S. Cochrane Database Syst Rev (3): CD004094

SECTION 11

1 Malkin CJ, Pugh PJ, Morris PD, Asif S, Jones TH, et al. Low serum testosterone and increased mortality in men with coronary heart disease. Heart. 2010;96:1821–5

2 Bach D, et al. "Long-term treatment of BPH. *Phytomed* 3 (1996): 105-11

3 Science. 1984 Sep 7;225(4666):1032-4

4 Urology. 2004 Apr;63(4):641-6

5 http://www.cancer.gov/ drugdictionary?cdrid=462587

SECTION 12

1 Lymphotoxin regulates commensal responses to enable diet-induced obesity. *Nature Immunology*, 2012; DOI: 10.1038/ ni.2403

2 A Hidden Trigger of Obesity: Intestinal Bugs, *Time*, Friday, Mar. 05, 2010, accessed online 3/2/2013, 744 pm, PST

3 *Br J Nutr.* 2008 Jun;99(6):1380-7. Epub 2007 Nov 22.

4 *Int J Obes.* 1984;8(4):289-93

5 *Dig Dis Sci.* 47 (8): 1697–704 Examples of vegetable gum fibers are guar gum and acacia Senegal gum.

6 J Nutr. 125 (6): 1401–1412

7 *J Nutr.* 137 (11 Suppl): 2527S–2533S

8 *J Nutr.* 137 (11 Suppl): 2563S–2567S

9 Jackson, Frank. "Breast Milk". Jackson GI Medical. http://www.prebiotin.com/ breast-milk/ Retrieved 16 June 2013

10 Int J Immunopathol Pharmacol. 2011 Jan-Mar;24(1 Suppl):45S-50S

11 Nature Reviews *Gastroenterology & Hepatology* volume 8, page 537 (2011)

12 Plant Foods Hum Nutr. 2018 Aug 31. doi: 10.1007/s11130-018-0689-7

13 Plant Foods Hum Nutr. 2017 Dec;72(4):418-424. doi: 10.1007/s11130-017-0643-0

14 http://www.superskinnyme.com/calories-in-cocktails.html

SECTION 13

1 Meier-Ewert HK, et al. Effect of sleep loss on C-reactive protein, an inflammatory marker of cardiovascular risk. J Am Coll Cardiol 2004;43(4):678-83

2 Donga E, et al. A single night of partial sleep deprivation induces insulin resistance in multiple metabolic pathways in healthy subjects. J Clin Endocrinol Metab. 2010;95(6):2963-8

3 Schmid SM, A single night of sleep deprivation increases ghrelin levels and feelings of hunger in normal-weight healthy men. J Sleep Res 2008 Sep;17(3):331-4

4 Spiegel K, et al. Impact of sleep debt on physiological rhythms. Rev Neurol (Paris. 2003;159(11 Suppl):6S11-20

5 Hogenkamp PS, et al. Acute sleep deprivation increases portion size and affects food choice in young men. Psychoneuroendocrinology 2013 Feb 18 (Epub ahead of print)

6 Reynolds AC, et al. Impact of five nights of sleep restriction on glucose metabolism, leptin and testosterone in young adult men. PLoS One 2012;7(7):e41218

7 Hursel R, et al. Effects of sleep fragmentation in healthy men on energy expenditure, substrate oxidation, physical activity, and exhaustion measured over 48 h in a respiratory chamber *Am J Clin Nutr* 2011;94(3):804-8

8 Van Cauter E, et al. Metabolic consequences of sleep and sleep loss. *Sleep Med* 2008;9 Suppl 1:S23-8

9 Chapman CD, et al. Acute sleep deprivation increases food purchasing in men. *Obesity* (Silver Spring). 2013 Aug 1

10 Gharib SA; Hayes AL; Rosen MJ; Patel SR. A pathway-based analysis on the effects of obstructive sleep apnea in modulating visceral fat transcriptome. SLEEP 2013;36(1):23–30

11 Sharma SK, Agrawal S, Damodaran D, Sreenivas V, Kadhiravan T, Lakshmy R, Jagia P, & Kumar A (2011). CPAP for the metabolic syndrome in patients with obstructive sleep apnea. *The New England Journal Of Medicine*, 365 (24), 2277-86

12 https://www.scientificamerican.com/article/supercharging-brown-fat-to-battle-obesity/

13 Rutin ameliorates obesity through brown fat activation. *Federation of American Societies for Experimental Biology Journal* (FASEB). Vol 31, no 1, January 2017

14 Obesity (Silver Spring). 2017 Jan;25(1):111-121. doi: 10.1002/oby.21706. Epub 2016 Nov 22

SECTION 14

1 European Congress on Obesity, news release, May 28, 2014

2 from the Mayo Clinic website: https://www.mayoclinic.org/healthy-lifestyle/nutrition-and-healthy-eating/in-depth/glycemic-index-diet/art-20048478

3 Nature volume 505, pages 559–563 (23 January 2014)

4 Lipids. 2009 Jul;44(7):593-601. doi: 10.1007/s11745-009-3306-6. Epub 2009 May 13

5 J Am Coll Cardiol. 2005 Nov 15;46(10):1864-8. Epub 2005 Oct 24

6 *The Journal of Nutrition*, Volume 130, Issue 2, 1 February 2000, Pages 272S–275S

7 historical notes from the HCG Diet Council: http://www.hcgdietcouncil.org/history-of-hcg-for-weight-loss/ accessed Aug 18th, 2013, 4.45 pm BST

8 Kathleen J. Melanson, Ph.D., R.D., L.D.N., associate professor, nutrition science, and director, Energy Balance Laboratory, University of Rhode Island, Kingston; Lona Sandon, R.D., assistant professor, clinical nutrition, University of Texas Southwestern, Dallas; abstract presented in November 2011, The Obesity Society annual meeting, Orlando, Fla.

SECTION 16

1 Fajnwaks P, Ramirez A, Martinez P, Arias E, Szomstein S, Rosenthal R (May 2008). “P46: Outcomes of bariatric surgery in patients with BMI less than 35 kg/m2”. *Surgery for Obesity and Related Diseases* 4 (3): 329

2 Snow V, Barry P, Fitterman N, Qaseem A, Weiss K (2005). “Pharmacologic and surgical management of this is not gastric bypass obesity in primary care: a clinical practice guideline from the American College of Physicians”. *Ann. Intern. Med.* 142 (7): 525–31

3 Robinson MK (July 2009). “Editorial: Surgical treatment of obesity—weighing the facts”. *N. Engl. J. Med.* 361 (5): 520–1

4 Maciejewski ML, Livingston EH, Smith VA, et al. (June 2011). “Survival among high-risk patients after bariatric surgery”. *JAMA* 305 (23): 2419–26

5 Chiles C, van Wattum PJ (2010). “Psychiatric aspects of the obesity crisis”. *Psychiatric Times* 27 (4): 47–51.

6 Tindle HA et al. Risk of suicide after long-term follow-up from bariatric surgery. *Am J Med* 2010 Nov; 123:1036

7 *JAMA Surg.* 2013;148(2):145-150. doi:10.1001/2013.jamasurg.26

8 *Science Translational Medicine* 27 Mar 2013: Vol. 5, Issue 178, pp. 178ra41 DOI: 10.1126/scitranslmed.3005687

9 Bacteria in the Intestines May Help Tip the Bathroom Scale, Studies Show, *New York Times*, March 27, 2013

SECTION 17

1 http:// www.mayoclinic.com/health/weight-loss-hypnosis/AN01617

SECTION 18

1 *Am J Clin Nutr.* 2005 Jul;82(1 Suppl):222S-225S

Index

A

B

C

D

E

F

Made in the USA
Monee, IL
24 October 2021